6·19·78

Parallel Play

a guide
to playground exercise

Parallel Play

a guide
to playground exercise

Eleanor Dinkin

Rosalind Urbont

Nelson Hall nh **Chicago**

Medical consultant: Leon G. Dinkin, MD, Mt. Sinai Hospital, New York; Modeling: Rosalind Urbont, Jack Urbont, Ariana Urbont, and Dawn Urbont; Drawing concepts and photography: Eleanor Dinkin

Library of Congress Cataloging in Publication Data

Dinkin, Eleanor.
  Parallel play

  Bibliography: p.
  Includes index.
  1. Exercise. 2. Playgrounds. I. Urbont,
Rosalind, joint author. II. Title.
  GV505.D5   613 7   78-23450
  ISBN 0-88229-424-5 (cloth)
  ISBN 0-88229-600-0 (paper)

Copyright © 1978 by Eleanor Dinkin and Rosalind Urbont

Manufactured in the United States of America

10 9 8 7 6 5 4 3 2 1

Contents

For Leon

Preface

In the exuberant and euphoric state of feeling fit as a fiddle, exercise enthusiasts are apt to promise everything. Exercise and the right approach to exercise will undoubtedly increase your feelings of well-being, of "vim, vigor, and vitality," but here is a word of caution.

Exercising regularly will *not* confer on you immortality, though conceivably it may add years to your life. It will *not* save your marriage if that is your problem, though conceivably feeling fit may make you better able to cope with problems. Regular exercise will *not* make your business boom, your career prosper, or your stocks go up, though feeling well may improve your business and professional judgment.

If approached with a sense of play and anticipation of enjoyment, exercising regularly will make you a healthier person, physically and emotionally. And really, isn't that enough?

It's helpful to exercise with someone else because it's more fun and it increases your commitment. It's not so easy to skip a day if you feel you're letting someone else down.

We were lucky. As neighbors with apartments on the same floor, we started exercising for half an hour every day. We exercised in the house and in the park; we talked, we read, and we gradually developed the ideas explored in this book. We were intrigued by the variety of exercise programs being taught and written about. This book grew naturally out of what we were doing as we clarified for ourselves the conflicting claims of different schools of thought. In Chapter 2, we explore the claims and counterclaims of the different exercise disciplines and the goals of physical fitness. In Chapter 3, we try to reconcile the seeming contradictions and to come out with a valid definition of a well-rounded exercise program.

We decided early in the writing of this book to try to bring some joy to the process of exercising, and this meant leaving the statisticians in the research laboratories. We don't believe you can enjoy exercising with a stopwatch in one hand, the fingers of your other hand on your pulse, your eyes on a table of levels, ages, and charts. At least you won't enjoy it for long. And, if you don't enjoy it, you'll soon drop it.

Statistics in themselves are descriptive of the average in a crowd of people but not necessarily individually valid or predictive. In our thinking we tend to substitute the word *norm* for *average* and *normal* for *norm*. Pretty soon, we begin to think that it's "abnormal" not to be average. The classic example: Try to be or to find the average (normal?) American family that, according to the latest census figures, has 1.9 children—literally, a family with one child and the mother 8.1 months pregnant with her second child. To try to conform to statistical averages is a futile endeavor and a meaningless preoccupation.

On the other hand, to realize that a British study[1] comparing London bus drivers (always sitting at the wheel and therefore sedentary) with London bus conductors (always standing, climbing up and down the stairs of the double decker buses, and therefore physically active) and finding that the bus conductors had

1. J. N. Morris, et al., "Coronary Heart Disease and Physical Activity of Work," *Lancet* Vol. 2, Nov. 21, 1953, pp. 1053-57.

fewer and less serious coronary problems is a meaningful piece of statistical research that has implications for all of us.

Aware of the effects of a sedentary life style for an otherwise healthy person, you can look into your own life and decide for yourself whether you should indeed be more active. The fact that you have read this far means that you have at least thought about exercising regularly. Perhaps you need only to find out how, and where and when.

Do these things and you are ready to begin.

1. Check with your physician. A medical checkup is a necessity before beginning any exercise program.

2. Make an exercise appointment with a friend. (It's more fun, and you'll feel less conspicuous exercising with a friend.)

3. Wear comfortable clothes and especially comfortable shoes.

4. Approach the whole problem of exercising with the idea that it's not a problem—it's a chance to be innovative and creative. Go to the park and enjoy yourself.

Our special thanks to Dr. Leon G. Dinkin, whose enthusiastic interest and moral support were as important to us as was his wise medical advice. He encouraged this project from the very beginning and saw it through to its final form and acceptance by our publisher.

We thank also Marjorie Stone for her valuable help in the editing process and Moshe Sheinbaum for generously sharing with us his knowledge of the publishing world.

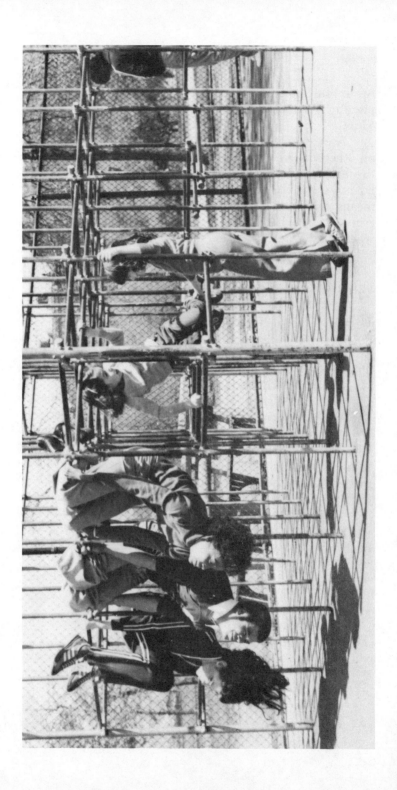

Chapter 1

Parallel
Play

How many times have you heard people say, "If only I had the time and the place to exercise every day"? This book is for those who already have the time and place to exercise but don't know it—for parents who take their young children to a playground for an hour or two every day and sit on a bench, chatting, reading, or just watching the children play. (The book may also be used by any adult who simply enjoys going to the park.)

If you are a parent who regularly visits a playground, did you ever stop to think that you don't have to watch from the sidelines? You don't have to fight boredom and figure out ways to kill time as you dutifully take your youngsters to the park. You don't have to look for other adults with whom to pass the time of day.

Your time at the playground can be productive, relaxing, and refreshing, and, above all, it can actively contribute to your physical well-being. The time is there. The equipment is there. Only the will is necessary. Instead of being a self-sacrificing parent (a questionable role to begin with), you can be a participating parent who finds as much enjoyment in this particular segment of the day's activities as the children do.

There is a great difference between the roles of the self-sacrificing parent and the participating parent, and between the meanings that these roles convey to the child at play.

1

Play is the child's way of relating to the world, of understanding the world, of testing himself in the world. Play is a very important part of his growth and maturation. The child at play is the child at work. To sit at the playground with a martyred expression and say, as some parents do, "Well, go and play now—you have an hour," is to degrade play and to express subtle disregard for it.

Imagine a woman saying to her husband, "Well, go and work now—you have seven hours." She doesn't say this. On the contrary, the husband is admired and rewarded for working. Too often the child is not. But an adult can let a child know that play is important by saying: "We're going to the playground. We'll both have an hour to play." An adult, too, needs to play—to test himself, to experience growth, to feel young.

Playing together does not always mean interacting. When very young children, two or three years old, first begin to function in a group, they play side by side, each in his own fantasy world. Psychologists call such activity *parallel play*.[1] An adult and a child who use the same

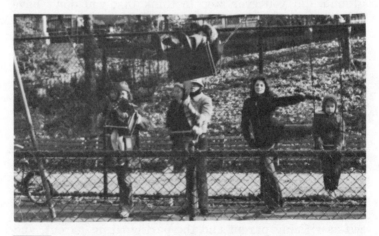

1. Susanna Millar, *The Psychology of Play* (Middlesex, Eng.: Penguin Books, 1968), p. 178.

equipment in the same period of time to satisfy different needs, and who "play" side by side, are actually involved in a kind of parallel play. The child swings; the adult exercises. What the adult is saying by this activity, in deeds rather than in words, is: "Play is important. I need to play too. Here we are, each doing his own thing. We're busy side by side—sometimes together, sometimes separately." That is the parallel play of adult and child which contributes to the growth of each.

We are concerned here with the adult at play because children don't have to be taught to play. Adults do. And if exercise is not play, is not fun, it will soon be dropped. Bud Wilkinson, the well-known coach and physical fitness adviser to President John Kennedy, has remarked: "The right kind of exercise not only is good for you, it's fun. ... I just don't believe that you're going to run in place in your bedroom for the rest of your life."[2] Neither do we. But what greater fun can there be than to play when your child is playing, to figure out ways to coordinate your activities with his, to reclaim time that was "lost" and to make it refreshing and productive? Going to the playground can be a time that you eagerly anticipate. This can be your parallel playtime. You can "play" with your children or alone or with other adults, depending on your mood and the mood and inclination of your child or children.

If you're embarrassed or hesitant to do this—to burst into activity in front of others at the park—don't be. You'll be setting the fashion. Some people who watch you will secretly want to do what you're doing but may be too shy. Others may take their cues from you. It is amazing how embarrassment disappears when you exercise with a friend. Don't be surprised if others join you. The more the merrier! As a group, you can plan a more

---

2. Bud Wilkinson, *Guide to Modern Physical Fitness* (New York: Viking, 1967), pp. 3, 4.

structured progression of exercises, if that is what you want.

Whether you work separately or with other parents, your child is your primary responsibility, and of course you'll always keep that special awareness of where your child is and what he is doing.

Chapter 2

The Language of Exercise

Different kinds of exercise seem to pass in and out of fashion like clothing styles. Fifty years ago there was great interest in calisthenics. Then came isometrics. In the early 1960s jogging became popular. In the late 1960s, aerobics was the thing to do. Later, yoga was the style. Today, the "in" exercise is again jogging.

The value of regular exercise for total well-being has been recognized since at least the time of the early Greeks. The great philosophers of early Greece stressed that only through physical activity and exercise could the body remain healthy and physically fit; they believed in the unity of body, mind, and spirit. The Greek ideal of education was expressed by Plato in his *Republic*: "Gymnastics as well as music should begin in early life; the training in it should be careful and should continue through life."[1] Exercise and gymnastics were an important part of the education of all Greek citizens. Of course, this was still an elitist approach since free citizens made up only 10 percent of the population. These free citizens —essentially idle because all labor and manual tasks were performed by the vastly larger slave population—had to find ways to stay in good physical condition. (The slave population had other problems and was not worried about exercising.)

---

1. Plato, *Republic*, Book III (New York: Random House, Modern Library Edition, 1934), p. 108.

In our modern Western industrial society, where
much of the hard labor and formerly manual tasks are
performed by machines, most of us are in the same position as the elite of ancient Greece: we have to find ways
to keep active and healthy. The very great current interest in the subject of exercise is the result. More than two
thousand years after Plato, a noted physiologist, Edward
C. Schneider, found it necessary to remark, "Frequently
repeated exercise, extending over months and years ... is
necessary for healthy existence; it is a physiologic need
of a primitive kind which cannot safely be eliminated by
civilization."[2]

Exercise is a word that comes originally from Latin:
ex, "out," and *arcere*, "to enclose." The term once meant
"to drive out from an enclosure" as animals to the fields
to work. The closest word in common usage today would
be *workout*, which is often used interchangeably with exercise. The words *practice* and *exercise* both denote repetitive actions; however, one practices in order to ac-
quire a specific skill, but one usually exercises in order
to develop some part of the body or for the improvement
of physical well-being. Exercise has a long term training
effect on an individual; the more a person exercises, the
longer he is able to exercise, and the more physically fit
he becomes.

But what does it mean to be physically fit? When a
person is physically fit, he performs his activities with
the least possible expenditure of effort due to a greater
efficiency of his cardiovascular system, to the increased
strength of his musculoskeletal apparatus, and to the
greater flexibility of his muscles and joints. Increased
physical fitness results in better balance, better coordination, a lower pulse rate, and a sense of well-being. According to Sir William Osler—a physician and professor

---

2. Charles A. Bucher, "You Still Need Exercise," *Today's Health*,
   Vol. 34, Dec. 1956, p. 24.

of medicine who practiced more than a century ago—low weight, low blood pressure, and especially low pulse rate are associated with maximum health. A physically fit person may also show greater resiliency and faster recovery from stress, fatigue, or even sickness. We agree also with the emphasis of the Royal Canadian Air Force Exercise Program on a personal assessment of fitness. "It [fitness] is how we feel when we get up in the morning; how tired or fresh we are after a hard day's work...."[3] Most writers on the subject consider physical fitness part of total fitness. (See section on Total Fitness in this chapter.)

What kinds of exercise should you use to become physically fit? In the reference volume *Subject Guide to Books in Print,* available at any public library, you can find hundreds of books listed under the headings Exercise, Gymnastics, Calisthenics, Yoga, Isometrics, and so on. All these books describe ways to exercise and stay healthy. Many make valid claims. Many make wild claims. Different methodologies are advocated; different beliefs are followed. Some books have religious overtones; some are scientific; some are pseudoscientific; some are personal testimonials.

The exercise beginner finds himself at sea, not knowing which course to chart through this verbal storm of claim and counterclaim. This book draws on different kinds of exercise, and so we thought it useful to describe the basic approaches to exercise—particularly their methods, goals, and claims—and to define the terms currently used in the field. We have tried to formulate the generally accepted meanings as briefly as possible but have expanded where we thought it appropriate and have digressed if we felt it necessary. The terms are in alphabetical order.

---

3. *Royal Canadian Air Force Exercise Plans for Physical Fitness,* rev. ed. (Ottawa, Can.: Crown Pub., 1962), p. 5.

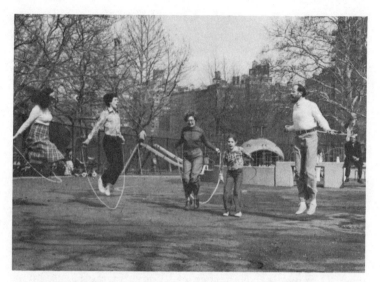

AEROBICS is an age-adjusted activity program re-
searched and developed by a major in the United States
Air Force, physiologist and physician Kenneth Cooper.
The original program, *Aerobics,* was first published in
1968, and the revised, age-adjusted program for the general public was published in 1970 under the title *The New
Aerobics.* By dictionary definition, the word *aerobic*
means "able to live, grow, or take place only where free
oxygen is present." Cooper uses the word to indicate
activities that increase oxygen consumption to the point
of speeding up the heart rate from the normal 72 to 76
beats per minute to 150 beats per minute for approximately five minutes. Aerobics favors regularly paced conditioning activities such as running, jogging, swimming,
rope jumping, and bicycling rather than unevenly paced
activities requiring short spurts of intensive effort—for
example, racing or other competitive sports.

Cooper has developed a system of assigning points
to various activities on the basis of their caloric require-
ments (the equivalent of the energy expended) as shown

in research data available in the medical literature. For example, he gives 1½ points to a twenty-minute set of singles (tennis) by players of equal ability. He also provides charts from which a person can determine the point value of a particular activity lasting for any specific length of time. According to this program, men must accumulate thirty points a week and women twenty-four points a week from any variety of these activities to achieve a beneficial effect. As a result of such "aerobic conditioning," the body gradually accommodates itself to more and more strenuous activity by increasing the capacity of the cardiovascular and pulmonary systems to deliver and to process oxygen.

Evidence is now accumulating to validate the positive effects of Cooper's approach. While the program appears to us to be complicated to follow and tedious in its use of charts and records, the basic theory of cardiac conditioning is obviously well founded.

CALISTHENICS is a term derived from two Greek words: *kallos*, "beauty," and *sthenos*, "strength." Calisthenics might therefore be defined as beauty through strength. It has come to mean simple exercises—for example, push-ups, sit-ups, and knee bends—done repeatedly for the purpose of developing a lean and strong body.

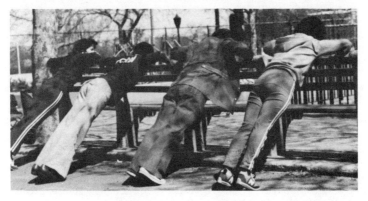

Progress is usually considered to consist of gaining the ability to do the exercises at a faster and faster pace in a shorter and shorter time and, to a degree, raising the heart rate, the respiration rate, and the perspiration rate. Done fast enough and long enough, calisthenics may produce some of the benefits of aerobics. The word *calisthenics* is sometimes used synonymously with the word *gymnastics*, but actually gymnastics is the broader term. Calisthenics is part of gymnastics, which includes such other categories of activities as acrobatics.

GYMNASTICS is also a word with Greek origins: *gymnos* means "naked" and *gymnazein* means "to train naked." From the latter term came *gymnasion*, a place where Greek citizens exercised naked. Greek gymnasiums were not only places where adults exercised, but were also renowned intellectual and social centers, a fact that illustrates the hierarchy of values of the ancient Greek culture. Plato wrote, "He who mingles music with gymnastics in the fairest proportions ... may he be rightly called the true musician and harmonist."[4]

Modern-day gymnastics developed in Sweden, Denmark, and Germany in the eighteenth and nineteenth centuries and was introduced into American education in the mid-nineteenth century. In its broadest meaning, gymnastics includes all exercises that can be performed in a gymnasium, with or without equipment. Such exercises include calisthenics, tumbling, acrobatics, and feats of skill. Gymnastics has often been associated in the public mind with various types of formal drills and as such seems to many to be militaristic and authoritarian in spirit. Modern-day educators in American public school systems tend to emphasize games, sports, and team activities as socially and politically more suitable for a democratic society.

---

4. Plato, *Republic*, Book III (New York: Random House, Modern Library Edition, 1934), p. 120.

ISOMETRICS is a term based on the Greek words *isos*, "equal," and *metron*, "measure," and indicates, generally, "equality of measure." Specifically in the field of exercise, isometrics denotes a type of exercise in which a set of muscles is tensed for a few seconds against an immovable object or against another equally tensed set of muscles. The basic principle on which isometrics is founded was actually discovered over fifty years ago in a laboratory experiment with frogs. The immobilized leg of a frog developed amazing strength through muscular tension as the frog struggled in vain to free itself. The importance of this discovery was overlooked for decades until two German physiologists, Theodor Hettinger and Erich A. Müller, realized its significance and did considerable research on the subject. In 1953, they published their findings in a German magazine and brought world attention to the value of isometrics in building strength in various muscles in extraordinarily short periods of time. For example, in pushing against an immovable object such as a wall for a few seconds, one works against an unconquerable resistance. Nothing moves, but the muscle tenses; its metabolism increases, and in time the muscle fibers become stronger and bigger.

Additional research in Europe and in the United States has attested to the value of isometrics in developing muscular strength, in therapeutically treating various kinds of injuries, and in developing proficiency in many fields of athletics. Isometrics has aroused widespread popular interest because the program can be practiced anywhere without the need for equipment and takes only a few minutes each day. Isometrics focuses mainly on muscular strength and does little to promote other important exercise objectives such as endurance, release of tension, and flexibility.

ISOTONIC EXERCISE. *Isotonic* derives from the Greek words *isos*, "equal," and *tonic*, "tension." In general usage, *isotonic* means "having equal tension." Specifically in the field of exercise, the term refers to a method of strengthening muscles by overcoming increasingly greater levels of resistance. For example, the lifting of progressively heavier weights is a form of isotonic exercise. Isometric exercises involve no movement, since the resistance cannot be overcome. All isotonic exercises involve movement as the resistance, whatever it is, is finally overcome. Isotonic exercises also include such traditional and familiar activities as calisthenics, acrobatics, push-ups, and all forms of gymnastics. These activities are all classical ways of strengthening specific sets of muscles in the musculoskeletal system. As with isometrics, they do little to condition the cardiovascular and respiratory systems unless they are performed with the intensity and persistence of such endurance activities as jogging and running.

JOGGING is a term derived from the Middle English *joggen*, "to spur a horse to movement." Generally,

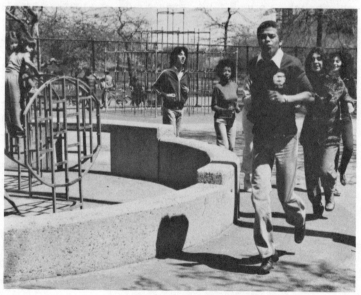

to jog means to shake or nudge a person to activity, mental or physical. In the field of exercise, the present participle *jogging* refers specifically to an evenly paced run or trot. Jogging became a popular and fashionable activity in the early 1960s because of President John Kennedy's interest in physical fitness. Who can forget the image of young Kennedy administrators, heaving and puffing as they jogged along a country road for the benefit of the press, fulfilling a presidential order to set the pace and style for national fitness? Probably more than any other president, Kennedy focused on the national need to keep healthy through activity. In many ways, jogging is the ideal activity. Suitable for groups or individuals, it requires no special equipment or setting and can be done in place, in a park, on a road. In 1967, W. J. Bowerman and W. E. Harris, M.D., wrote *Jogging*, a book that formalized jogging with schedules and three-day-a-week formulas suited to the age and fitness of the individual. Jogging in place, or "stationary running," rates high on Cooper's aerobic charts. Today, jogging has the further advantage of providing a partial answer to the problems of energy, transportation, and inflation. Jog to work and you save money and conserve fuel while becoming more physically fit.

PHYSICAL CULTURE is a phrase that came into use in the late 1800s to denote courses in the culture of the body as opposed to courses in the culture of the soul and of the intellect. The term was later popularized by Bernarr MacFadden and other businessmen in very successful commercial enterprises promoting health through exercise.

The sales pitch of some of the less scrupulous companies echoed the spiel of the medicine peddlers of the old time West. ("One dollar a bottle. Cures all human diseases.") Now the phrase brings to mind the "physical culture nut" with his extravagant claims and scorn for all medical opinion.

PHYSICAL TRAINING refers to those activities—
such as exercise, muscular work, and participation in
sports—that would lead a sedentary, inactive person
from a poor physical condition to a trained, or physically
fit, condition. A person in a trained condition of course
functions more efficiently with less expenditure of
energy. In order for physical training to be effective, it
must suit a person's age and physical condition; it must
be practiced on a fairly regular basis (you can't store
training as a camel stores water); and the activity must
be lengthy enough and intense enough to obtain a specific
physiological response. The benefits of training are
cumulative.

SLIMNASTICS is a word coined by two British
women, Pamela Nottidge and Diana Lamplugh, and the
title of their book on figure improvement. Basically, Slimnastics is a social approach to exercise and diet. The system somewhat resembles that of Weight Watchers but
includes exercise as well as diet. Nottidge and Lamplugh
have devised their own graded exercise schedules for five
age levels. The exercises are a hybrid of calisthenics and
yoga. For those who would like to exercise indoors in a
group but who do not want to pay salon prices, this approach may be the answer. For people who need help in
organizing such a group, we recommend Chapter 5 of
Nottidge and Lamplugh's book.

TAI CHI is a classical Chinese exercise system developed to train the Kung Fu warriors of ancient China.
Some of its present-day adherents make extravagant
claims for its therapeutic, medicinal, and spiritual benefits, and it has been surrounded by a cultish mystique for
years. The titles of the Tai Chi exercises, or postures,
add to this mystique—for example, "Touch the South
Wind," "The Sun Wheel," "Bird with Folded Wing,"
and "Dark Lady Spins Flax."

Tai Chi is actually a series of intricate postures, not exercises. The postures, which are not so extreme as those of Hatha Yoga, involve only natural body movements that flow into one another. Some of the instructions, such as "body is turned to face East," can obviously have no physiological effect; but the total concentration required in memorizing the detailed instructions is said to produce relaxation. Implausible claims aside, practice of Tai Chi is said to promote eye-limb coordination, flexibility, relaxation, and balance. The postures have little or no effect on cardiovascular conditioning or development of muscular strength.

TOTAL FITNESS is a broad concept that indicates fitness in physical, emotional, mental, and social functioning—that is, all the ways in which one functions as an effective, integrated, mature, and healthy person. Leonard Gross and Lawrence Morehouse popularized the expression as the title of their book on exercise and diet published in 1975. Actually, their book deals only with physical fitness.

Gross and Morehouse define physical fitness in terms of cardiovascular efficiency, and therefore they concern themselves with ways to increase this efficiency. They suggest performing exercises—even for a few minutes a day—in such a way that the exertion temporarily increases the heart rate, thereby strengthening the heart muscle and promoting the efficiency of the entire system. Such gains are evidenced, eventually, by a lower pulse rate at rest and during exercise. Cooper takes the same basic approach in his aerobics program.

Gross and Morehouse then turn to the questions of how much exercise is necessary: what is enough and what is too much. They describe the results of research done at the National Aeronautics and Space Administration (NASA) on the problem of designing exercise programs specifically for astronauts. A low-gravity situation, such as the astronauts find in space, sharply reduces the amount of effort needed to complete a task. Under these conditions, doing a certain number of exercisés does not guarantee that the body is getting the amount of exercise it needs. The designers of the NASA program therefore began to disregard performance per se and to concentrate on the amount of physical exertion required for performance. They used the pulse rate as the indicator of this exertion and called it "the marvelous computer." By exercising until his pulse reached a predetermined rate, an astronaut could be sure he was exerting himself enough to stay in shape—on earth, in space, or on the moon.

But we are still on earth and will, no doubt, remain here. Gross and Morehouse basically agree with Cooper and suggest exercising until your pulse reaches a specific rate for a given period of time. They include in their book various schedules, tables, and formulas to help you find your pulse rate goals. As with Cooper's plan, as a general guide to conditioning this program seems feasible if not taken too rigidly, and if not turned into a bookkeeping procedure.

XBX AND 5BX are two exercise plans developed by the Royal Canadian Air Force (RCAF). XBX is a twelve-minute-a-day plan for women. A team of RCAF specialists developed it over a period of two years, and more than six hundred women participated in the research program. The plan consists of four charts, each listing ten exercises. Nine of the exercises on each chart are of the calisthenic type, and the tenth is a variation on jogging. The charts are arranged in a series that becomes progressivly more difficult. There are forty-eight levels of fitness, and one goes at one's own pace as far as age and physical condition allow. The plan involves chart watching, time checking and daily record keeping of performance and timing. Like other statistically oriented exercise programs, it necessitates exercising with stop-watch in one hand, pencil and paper in the other and an eye on the charts. Some people thrive on it; others find it tedious.

5BX, the companion eleven-minute-a-day exercise plan for men, was also developed on the basis of RCAF research. This plan consists of six charts, each listing five exercises, and a thirty-level plan to attain physical fitness. Our comments about XBX apply also to 5BX.

YOGA is an ancient Hindu discipline practiced for centuries in India and enjoying a revival in the United States today. The Sanskrit word *yoga* means "union," and the goal was union with a universal soul or life-force known as *prana.* Yoga, taught by wise men, or *gurus,* included two main disciplines, Raja Yoga and Hatha Yoga.

Raja Yoga has to do with meditation and is the source of the currently popular transcendental meditation movement (TM). Legend has it that ancient gurus lived on mountaintops in seclusion and poverty, and their disciples traveled hundreds of miles on foot to see them. Modern-day gurus appear on TV and may be heads of multinational corporations!

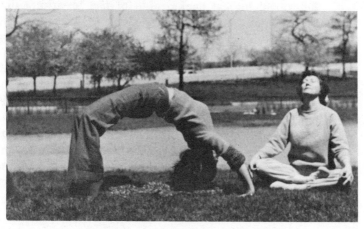

Hatha Yoga includes the physical aspect of this ancient discipline; when people speak of yoga exercise, they mean Hatha Yoga. Such exercise is practiced today by people who do not necessarily accept the philosophic, religious, or cultish implications of Raja Yoga. Strictly speaking, Hatha Yoga is not a series of exercises but a system of intense inner concentration, controlled breathing, and slow stretching and holding after reaching any one of the basic eighty-four postures or *asanas* (some of which are extremely difficult). The physical goals are the development of a healthy and supple body; the relief of tension and stiffness; the development of a flexible spine; and the cultivation of a sense of tranquility. Many people who practice Hatha Yoga testify to the personal benefits experienced.

There is nothing mysterious or mystical about this. The slow stretching and holding of difficult positions often require the use of muscles and joints that have not been sufficiently exercised for years. The fibers of the muscles and the ligaments of the joints are lengthened and strengthened by this process, resulting in the flexible spine and the suppleness of joints that Hatha Yogis talk about.

The physiological background of the breathing discipline is understood now as a fight to overcome the chemical effects of hyperventilation, which is always present to some degree when people are tense. Such hyperventilation has its roots in an ancient reflex of all animals, including man, to react to danger with a preparation for "fight or flight." In such a situation, a person overbreathes so as to store reserve oxygen. Ordinarily, people today don't physically fight or flee, and the extra oxygen remaining in the body causes unpleasant feelings through alkalosis—a chemical imbalance in the bloodstream. Therefore, regulated, slow breathing is very helpful in releasing tension and in promoting tranquility.

Chapter 3

The Plan
of Exercise

We hope it has become apparent that the different exercise approaches do not conflict with one another but, instead, promote a variety of objectives, all of which are important in the overall fitness concept. In advocating one particular approach, it is not necessary to tear down and rip apart all other approaches; yet that is precisely what is done in the field of exercise today.

For example, one well-known authority on yoga states that the benefits of Hatha Yoga "far surpass those of any system of self-improvement for the body (calisthenics, salon programs, jogging, isometrics, competitive sports)...."[1] Later in the same work, he writes, "Inherent in most systems of calisthenics is the need to execute many quick repetitions of the exercises; huff, puff, perspire and experience general discomfort and fatigue...."[2]

With an opposite view, an authority on aerobics quotes one of his students: "No exercise has the stuff, unless it makes you huff and puff."[3] He writes about isometrics: "These are superficial frame muscle manipulators that can leave you overstressed, trembling, unper-

1. Richard Hittleman, *Yoga 28 Day Exercise Plan* (New York: Workman, 1969), p. 9.
2. Ibid., p. 42.
3. Roy Ald, *Jogging, Aerobics, and Diet* (New York: Signet Books, 1968), p. 39.

spired, and unimproved. . . . For someone who can get up
and get around and do better, 'for shame.' "[4]

The aerobic approach concentrates on effort. "Unless the exercise is of sufficient intensity and duration it
will not produce a training effect and cannot be classified
as an aerobic exercise."[5]

It is obvious that Hatha Yoga would be rated zero
on the aerobic scale of effort. Is Hatha Yoga worth nothing then? Not at all. It has different goals, equally important. Hatha Yoga concentrates on flexibility of spine
and suppleness of joints as well as an overall feeling of
tranquility. Aerobics would probably rate zero on a
Hatha Yoga scale if there were one. Aerobics concentrates on increasing effort in order to condition the heart
and respiratory system.

On an aerobic scale, calisthenics would probably be
rated according to speed of performance, effort expended, and duration of activity. But on our imaginary
yoga scale, calisthenics would most likely be rated on the
basis of slowness and the amount of stretching and holding that was done. Isometrics would most likely rate zero
on both a yoga scale and an aerobics scale: isometrics
focuses specifically on developing muscular strength.

Well, where do we go from here? To whom do we
listen? Throw out everything, the baby with the bath
water, and start over? Not at all.

We feel there is a valid comparison between the sub-
jects of healthful exercise and healthful diet. A healthful
diet is a well-balanced one that provides enough varieties
of foods—including proteins, carbohydrates, and fats—
to supply all the different nutritional needs of the body.
Such a diet is appropriate for most people. There are
problems, obviously, that require special diets, but generally, a well-rounded, balanced diet is considered a
sound health practice.

---

4. Ibid., p. 38.
5. Kenneth H. Cooper, MD, *The New Aerobics* (New York: Bantam Books, 1970), p. 16.

We believe also that a healthful exercise program should have enough variety in the kinds of exercise to satisfy all the different fitness needs of the body. Such a program would keep the body functioning as efficiently as possible and also slow down the processes of aging—the often unspoken goal of all exercise programs. We believe a well-rounded exercise program should include various categories of activities. For conditioning heart and lungs, there should be such endurance exercises as jogging, running, or fast-paced calisthenic activity. For strengthening muscles, there should be isometric or other specific exercises aimed at target areas. There should be stretching exercises, such as those of yoga, to promote suppleness of joints and flexibility of spine. Finally, there should be some controlled breathing techniques as in yoga to promote the ability to consciously release tension; such techniques, together with the other activities, would promote a feeling of well-being.

These goals are really nothing more than different components of physical fitness that have been studied for years and cataloged in various research articles. What we have done is to work backwards from the desirable goals to the selection of exercise approaches that are aimed at these goals as stated by the proponents themselves.

Finally, this simple but important concept emerges: *A well-rounded exercise program should include moderate amounts of different kinds of exercise such as yoga, isometrics, calisthenics, and endurance-type activities which would lead a sedentary, inactive person from a poor physical condition to a physically fit or trained condition.*

It now becomes clear that it is not at all necessary to choose only one form of exercise—yoga or calisthenics or isometrics or aerobics. To continue with our diet analogy, that would be like choosing to eat only carbohydrates or only proteins. In the well-rounded exercise program, a variety of kinds of activities leads simultaneously to the fulfillment of various needs and goals.

Illustrated Basic Concept of a Well-Rounded Exercise Program

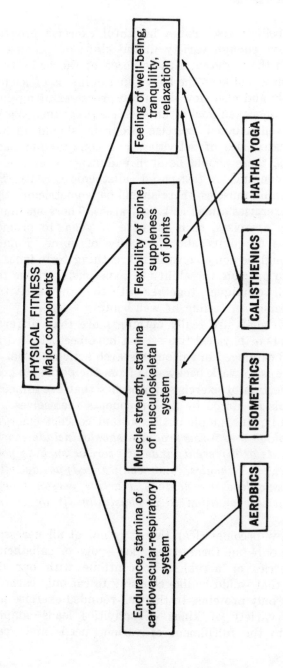

Types of exercise approaches with arrows pointing to their major goals.

There is also another aspect that we have not yet touched on: boredom. It would be boring to eat only carbohydrates, day in and day out. It is also boring to do only one kind of exercise, day in and day out. In fact, boredom may be the major reason why many people begin exercise programs with enthusiasm and drop them with relief.

Therefore, we have tried to design our parallel play exercise program to provide variety and have purposely included four fundamental types of exercise at each piece of equipment used in this program. We have selected the basic equipment found in most playgrounds—swings, jungle gym, seesaw—and also the park bench. Because

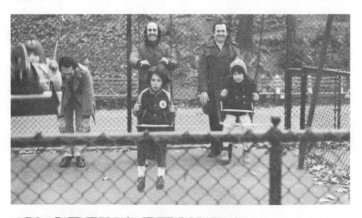

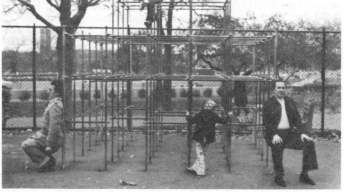

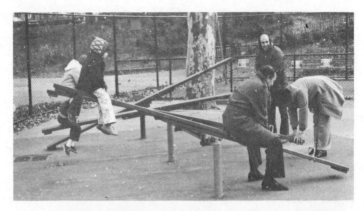

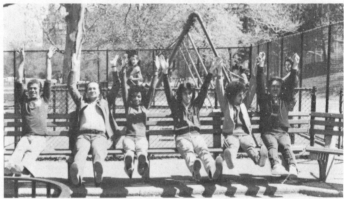

this book is intended primarily for parents of young
children, we have developed a series of exercises that can
be done in coordination with the activities of an active,
not always predictable, child. If your child has taken a
liking to one apparatus, as children sometimes do, you
can stay there the whole time that you are at the playground, and you will still have a balanced exercise program. On the other hand, if your child wants to go from
one apparatus to another with you, you can do isometrics
at one, calisthenics at another, yoga stretches and breathing exercises at a third, and endurance-type exercises
anywhere. And, finally, if your child wants to go freely

off by himself into his world of children and play, you don't have to feel deserted! You can play parallel! There are several series of exercises that you can do by yourself to achieve a balanced program encompassing four fundamental types of exercise. They may be done at the bench, at the seesaw (using it as a slantboard), at the jungle gym (using it as a ballet bar), or even without any equipment.

So too, if you want to concentrate on only one target —for example, abdominal exercises for postpartum mothers—well, do this; but when you've achieved your goal, start balancing your program. A narrowed routine for certain specific purposes may be desirable for a limited time, but not forever. The goal of any good exercise program should be that state of physical fitness that promotes optimum functioning in all areas of activity.

How much exercise, and how to begin? First of all, we repeat, before you start any exercise program, check with your physician to determine what amount of activity is particularly good for you and if there are any restrictions. But after that, your goals can be personally set and personally evaluated. If you can't touch the floor in the touch toe exercises, to do so will become your goal.

We think that in all the activities except those of the endurance type, you must set your own goals because only you know yourself. For example, you know how much you need to relax. You know whether or not you tend to hyperventilate and can, therefore, determine how much practice in controlled breathing you need. You know if you can reach the yoga-type postures easily or have to work each day to do a little more. For endurance-type activities, such as jogging or fast-paced calisthenics, it may be a good idea to be aware of the standards set by a tested program such as the Royal Canadian Air Force Exercise Plan described under the heading "XBX and 5BX" in Chapter 2. Alternatively, the theories of aerobics and other pulse rating systems may be helpful. All these plans aim to strengthen the cardiovascular and pulmonary systems through exercising, at least for a few minutes, with a racing pulse. Whether you exercise at a pulse rate of 150 beats per minute, as advocated in Cooper's Aerobics program, or use Gross and Morehouse's Total Fitness formulas is up to you and to your physician to decide.

How should you evaluate the results of exercising? Again, we prefer the personal approach: only you yourself known how you feel, whether you are improving, what you can begin to do that you couldn't do before, and whether you have increased your feeling of well-being. If, however, you want a more objective way of evaluating your improvement in overall stamina, you may check your resting pulse rate after a month to see if you have lowered it. If you are a point-and-figure person and like to keep numerical records of progress, then look into the aerobics program and evaluate your activities by Cooper's point grading system. We believe that it is both possible and desirable to learn something from every system and approach.

Sometimes it doesn't hurt to state the obvious. Before proceeding any further we would like to emphasize that playgrounds were developed for children; we are very much aware of that. In the context of this book and

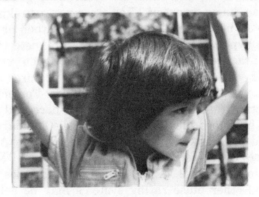

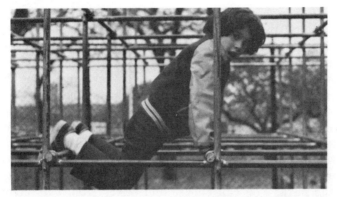

the program that we are recommending, we feel we must state that any piece of equipment should be used by an adult only if children are not using it. The image of an anxious adult rushing to grab a place at the seesaw before a four-year-old gets there is definitely not appealing, neither to us nor, we are sure, to the readers! However, this does not rule out adult activity. If you wander into any park during the daytime hours when parents take their children to the playground, you will probably see that a great deal of equipment is idle, and you will have your choice of what to use. If everything is in use, there are still the bench exercises, which encompass a balanced exercise program. Having said this and cleared our conscience, we can proceed.

The plan here consists of designing a variety of exercises for the basic kinds of equipment found in most playgrounds and for the park bench found almost everywhere. In the next chapter, "Bench Warm-ups," we start off with some very simple warm-up exercises and stretches, which should take only two or three minutes. In the ninth chapter, "Back to the Bench," we have more vigorous exercises for use at the bench when all other equipment has been preempted. Chapter 9 also includes a section on rope jumping, which may of course be done almost anywhere in a park.

In summary, our main purpose is to invite you
to use and to make the most of the playground and its
equipment and of the time that you ordinarily spend
there, to invite you to "play parallel" with your child as
soon as you get to the park. After you have gone over the
suggestions outlined here, we recommend that you look
around at your own particular environment and recog-
nize new opportunities for parallel play and exercise. We
present the following chapters, not as recipes to be followed rigidly, but rather as a menu of a whole variety of
possibilities that present themselves to you when you go
to the park. You can choose and select from this menu
and also modify it to your own tastes, needs, and goals.

Chapter 4

Bench
Warm-ups

You can begin exercising the moment you sit down on a park bench. This is where you start warming up. In sports, warm-ups are preparatory exercises that athletes perform before going into the big game or athletic contest. Such exercises are done to increase circulation, to loosen tight muscles and joints—in short, to "rev" up the body for the more vigorous activity to come.

Children don't need a warm-up phase when they come to the park to play. They are usually in constant physical motion wherever they are. Their bodies are young and flexible, and they can plunge into the playground activities without any difficulties. In a sense, they are warming up from the moment they awaken in the morning. A college athlete was scheduled to go through all the motions that a two-year-old child did in one day; after only a few hours, the athlete felt completely exhausted. We need not be concerned about preparing children for physical activity at the playground.

It is quite another story for adults. Adults are more sedentary than children; their joints are not as flexible; their muscles are often unused and taut; they generally look for ways to conserve energy rather than to expend it. Adults need a gradual transition to any activities more strenuous than their usual daily routines. The exercises in this chapter are designed to provide such a transition.

Their objectives are to limber you up, to relax and stretch tight muscles, to gradually increase the intensity of your activity, and so to ease you into the process of exercising.

In addition, a warm-up phase has certain psychological advantages for exercising in the park. It is somehow easier to start exercising inconspicuously, sitting where you usually sit. Also, if you want others to exercise with you, the bench is the best place to start. It's like going into the ocean slowly; the bench is the place where you get your feet wet, so to speak.

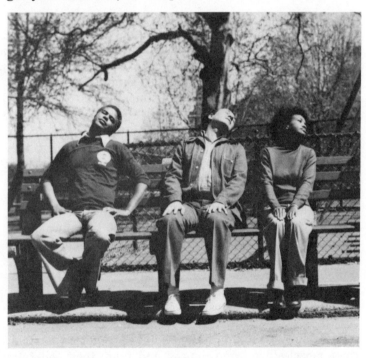

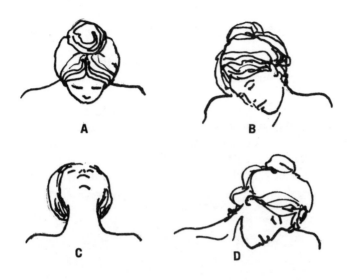

Head Roll

1. Sit erect on bench.
2. Place hands on knees.
3. Drop head forward, chin resting against chest (A).
4. Roll head very slowly in complete circular motion. (B, C, D).
5. Return to starting position, chin on chest (A).
6. Repeat in opposite direction (A, D, C, B, A).
7. Repeat slowly, three times in each direction, each time making wider and wider circles, slowly S-T-R-E-T-C-H-I-N-G neck muscles.

Target: neck muscles

Comment: This is a yoga-derived exercise, referred to by yogis as the Neck Roll, although obviously it is the head that rolls and the neck that stretches!

Bench Stretch

1. Sit up straight, hands at your sides holding bench (A).
2. Slowly raise and extend left leg, stretching leg as far as possible and drawing circle in air with left ankle (B). Think S-T-R-E-T-C-H as you do it.
3. Gradually relax left leg and return to position (A).
4. Do the same exercise with right leg (C).
5. Now slowly raise both legs simultaneously and also raise both arms high above head, stretching as you do this (D). Draw circles with wrists and

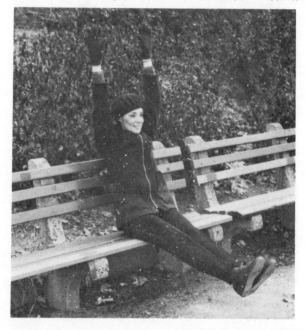

   ankles for a count of ten. Feel S-T-R-E-T-C-H as you do this.
6. Ease back into original position (A).

Target: arms and legs

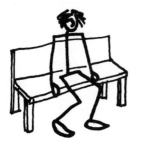

A

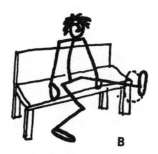

B

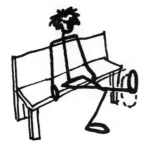

C

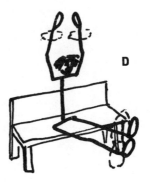

D

33

Deep Breathing

1. Sit on bench, hands on knees, back straight. Exhale completely.
2. Contract abdomen, pushing any residual air out of lungs.
3. Inhale very slowly, expanding abdomen and then raising shoulders, thus giving lungs maximum space to expand.
4. Hold breath for count of five.
5. Exhale slowly, lowering shoulders and contracting abdomen.
6. Repeat three times.

Target: relaxation

Comment: Why teach breathing when you've been breathing all your life without any conscious effort or help from anyone? Breathing is an autonomic function: a baby starts breathing without any instructions. However, some people tend to overbreathe, bringing on the symptoms of hyperventilation. Practice in slow, deep breathing releases tension and helps prepare you for exercising properly.

Rag Doll Shakes

1. Stand in front of bench.
2. Begin to shake your arms from the shoulders down as though you were a rag doll and someone were shaking you.
3. At the same time, let your head flop forward and allow it to shake and gently roll.
4. While continuing these movements, shake first your right leg and then your left leg; continue to shake legs alternately (A).

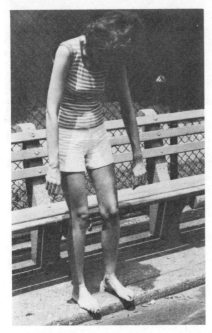
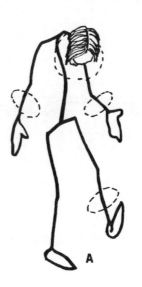

2037492

Target: limbering up

Comment: About one minute of this activity should give you a greater feeling of looseness and flexibility and prepare you for exercising.

Accelerated Bench Walk

1. Stand in front of bench.
2. Walk slowly around bench.
3. The second time you circle bench, break into a slow run.

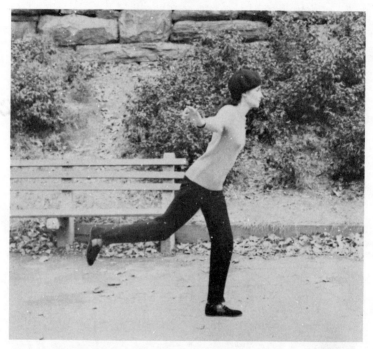

4. Increase pace and begin leaping (A). Each time you leap, imagine that you are hurdling a puddle of water.
5. Accelerate into a fast run and circle bench two or three times. Your children may love to do this entire exercise with you, especially if you turn it into a game of Follow the Leader.

Target: cardiovascular warm-up

Comment: Obviously, you do not have to walk around the bench if that is not convenient, but gauge the distance you walk before changing pace to the approximate distance around the bench. About one minute of this activity is all you need to gradually increase the rhythm of your cardiovascular and respiratory systems so that you are warmed up and ready for the next phase of exercising—whether it is at the swings, the seesaws, the jungle gym, or back to the bench.

Chapter 5

Variations
on a Swing

When you push your child in the swing, you will notice that you develop a natural rhythm for pushing in coordination with the rhythm of the moving swing. It goes something like this. Push. Wait (as the swing goes and returns). Push. Wait. Push. Wait. Notice that the waiting interval is somewhat longer than the pushing interval. The swing is actually a pendulum, and the time that it takes to go and to return is a function of the length of the chains of the swing, the weight of your child, the energy of your push, and gravity! Without going into complicated mathematical formulas, it is sufficient to note here that, since there are variables involved, *everyone's swinging time will be different.* Push your child on the swing three or four times and become aware of your own natural rhythm. Count if it helps. "Push, 2, 3, 4, push, 2, 3, 4, . . ." In the waiting interval, be aware of what you are doing. Usually one just stands there, fiddling, chatting, or daydreaming. Our objective here is to make use of this waiting time and, within the framework of the natural rhythm of pushing your child on the swing, to begin parallel exercise.

As you go through the following exercises, you may find that your particular waiting interval is not long enough to complete an activity. If so, simply change your rhythm to extend this interval. Instead of pushing

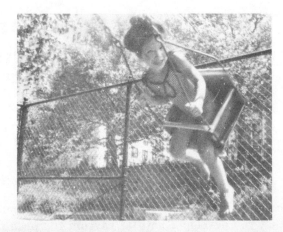

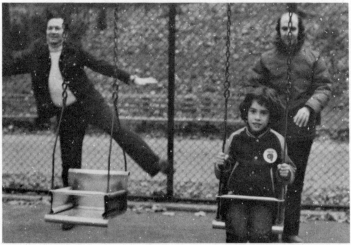

every return of the swing, push every other return of
the swing, giving you a rhythm something like this:
"Push, 2, 3, 4, 5, 6, push, 2, 3, 4, 5, 6 . . ."

You probably won't be able to do all the exercises the
first day. After all, it will depend not only on how fast
you master them but also on how much your child likes
swinging! We do not recommend pressuring your child

to stay on the swing any longer than he wants to. He may, however, be delighted with what you are doing, feel that the activity is something "special," and really enjoy swinging longer than usual. You will have to determine this as you go along. You will probably be able to do at least two or three of these exercises each time you go to the park and, if you perform them regularly, you will become more and more skillful at them.

Before each exercise, push the swing a few times to start the natural rhythm into which you work the exercise. Now you can begin the parallel play: your child swinging and you exercising!

Windmill

1. Push swing. At conclusion of push, arms will be extended (A, page 42).
2. Move extended arms like the giant blades of a windmill: upward, backward, downward, and forward to starting position (B, C, D, A).

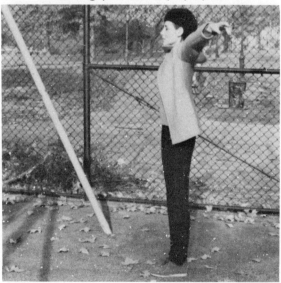

3. When swing returns, push it again and then repeat windmill movement.
4. Repeat five times.
5. The next time swing returns, push it and move
   both arms in reverse direction (D, C, B, A).
6. Repeat five times.

Target: arms, shoulders, and neck

   Comment: Do this exercise slowly, S-T-R-E-T-C-H-I-N-G
arms as you go through the circular windmill movements.
This exercise is aimed at releasing tension in the shoulder
and neck areas.

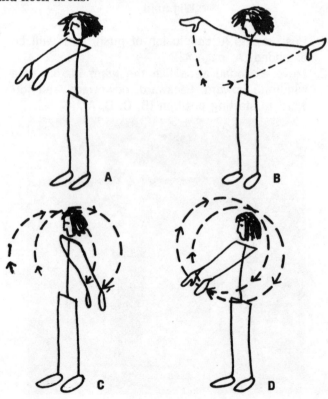

Swing Stretch

1. Push swing (A, page 44).
2. Kick left foot up, trying to touch extended left arm (B).

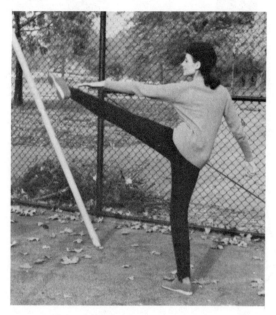

3. Hold position and S-T-R-E-T-C-H until swing reaches its peak.
4. As swing returns, return to starting position (A).
5. Repeat, this time kicking right foot up to try to touch extended right arm.
6. Do five times, alternating feet.

Target: abdomen and thighs

Comment: This exercise is aimed at strengthening and firming the abdominal muscles and the muscles of the upper legs.

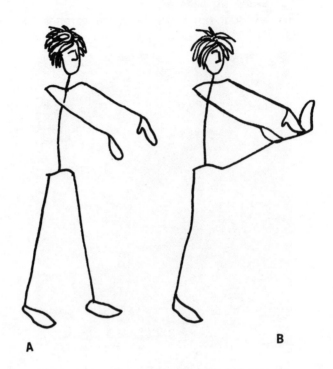

A   B

Variation: Side Swing Stretch

1. Push swing.
2. Extend right arm sideways; simultaneously kick right foot sideways trying to touch extended right arm (A, page 45).
3. As swing returns, return to starting position.
4. Push swing again, this time extending left arm sideways and kicking left foot sideways trying to touch extended left arm (B, page 45).

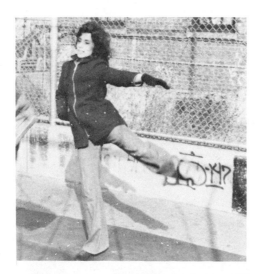

5. As swing returns, return to starting position.
6. Repeat five time, alternating right and left sides.

Target: waist and thighs

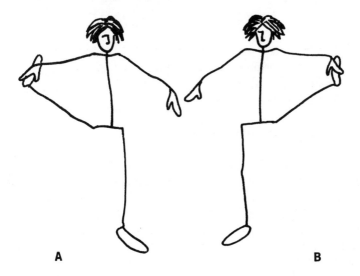

A   B

Touch Toe Stretch

1. Stand erect, feet a few inches apart. Push swing (A).
2. Bend and touch toes without bending knees (B).

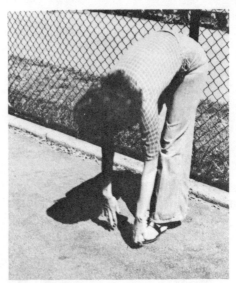

3. Straighten up, hands on hips (C).
4. Extend arms forward to meet returning swing and push again (A).
5. Repeat five times.

Target: back and thighs

Comment: If you can't yet touch your toes, then just bend down as far as you can go, keeping your legs straight. This is a good exercise for slowly stretching those tight muscles in your spine. If you practice this regularly, you may be able to touch not only your toes, but also the ground and even to place the palms of your hands on the ground.

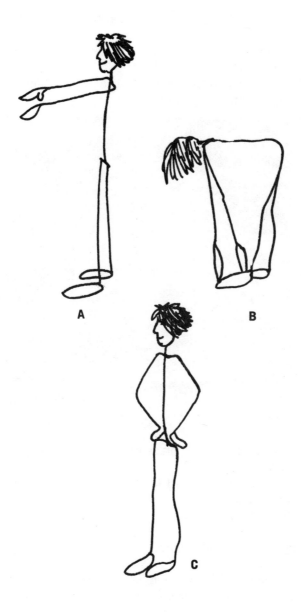

A

B

C

Variation: **Touch Toe Stretch**

1. Stand erect with feet at least two feet apart. Push swing (A).
2. Bend and touch ground between your feet without bending knees (B).

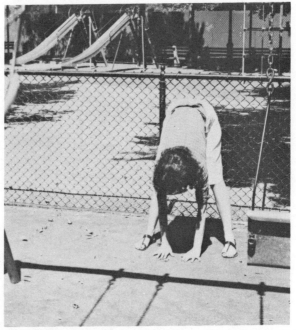

3. Straighten up and place hands on hips. Keep feet two feet apart (C).
4. Extend arms forward to meet returning swing and push again (A).
5. Repeat five times.

Target: back and thighs

Comment: This position helps stretch not only the muscles of the spine but also the muscles of the legs and upper thighs.

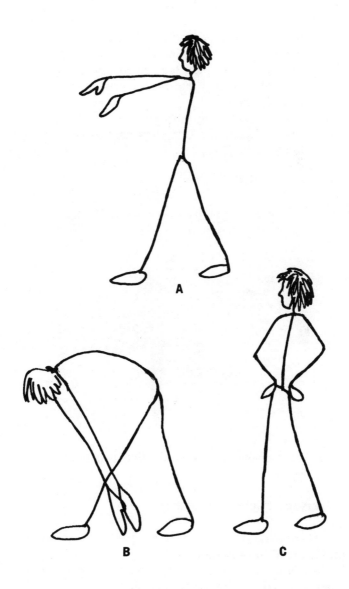

A

B

C

Palm Tree

1. Stand erect, feet together, hands by sides.
2. Bend right leg, bringing right heel to rest on left front thigh (A). Feel tension in upper leg.
3. Maintain position and push swing from this position two times.
4. Return to starting position.
5. Bend left leg and bring left heel to rest on right front thigh (B).

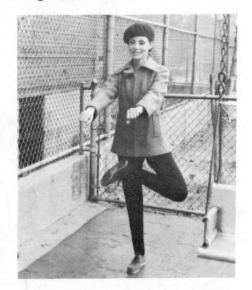

6. Push swing from this position two times.
7. Relax.

Target: thighs and balance

Comment: This exercise is aimed at firming the leg muscles and improving balance and coordination. As your balance improves, increase the number of times that you push the swing from each position.

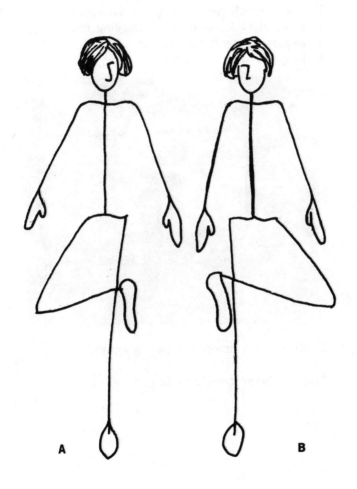

A B

Knee Hug

1. Stand erect, feet together. Push swing.
2. Bring right knee to chest, hugging folded leg.
3. Release leg and push swing.
4. Hug left knee to chest.

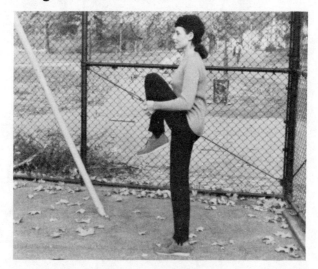

5. Repeat ten times, alternating knees.

Target: lower back and thighs

Sky Stretch

1. Push swing.
2. Stand on toes, raising arms toward sky (A).

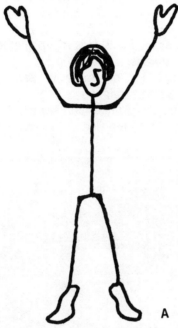

A

3. Hold and S-T-R-E-T-C-H. Reach for the tops of the trees, or the clouds, or whatever you see up there.
4. Return to starting position to meet returning swing.
5. Repeat five times.

Target: relaxation of tight muscles

Swing Squeeze

After your child has finished swinging, or while he swings alone, you can do the Swing Squeeze, using the structure of the swing for this isometric exercise.

1. Stand between two legs of upside-down frame at side of swings.
2. Grasp one leg of frame in each hand, palms inward, arms straight.
3. Try (unsuccessfully of course) to bring your hands together. Hold for five or six seconds (A).

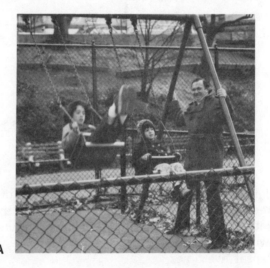

A

Target: arms, shoulders, and back

Comment: A variation of this exercise is to place the palms of your hands on the inside of the frame and push outward. In this way you use a slightly different set of muscles. Use whichever variation you feel best doing.

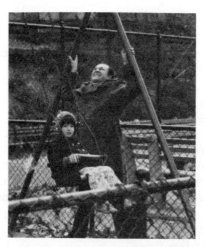

If either exercise is repeated each time you go to the park, over a period of months the resultant strengthening of your arms and back will be gratifying. Of course, the results depend also on how much you put into the exercise. If you exert only light pressure, you'll experience only mild strengthening. If you can manage an intense effort, even for two or three seconds at a time, you may have results that will surprise you. Like everything else, it's up to you.

Imaginary Girdle

This isometric exercise can also be done while your child swings by himself.

1. Stand straight, heels together, toes about six inches apart.
2. Place hands on thighs and bend trunk forward, bending elbows as you do.
3. In bent position, contract abdominal muscles intensely. (Imagine you are wearing a girdle that is too tight for you.) Hold for a few seconds.
4. Relax and do some deep breathing as described in Chapter 4.
5. Repeat five times.

Target: abdomen

Comment: As with all isometrics, the benefits accrued depend on the intensity of your efforts during that short hold of a few seconds. If you are in bad shape, we suggest that you build up your efforts gradually over a period of days or even weeks. If you want to feel what you are doing, place one hand on your stomach as you do the "hold" in step 3. Feel the wall of your abdomen stiffen as your muscles tighten. Do only a few seconds a day. Over a period of weeks, you will begin to notice that your stomach muscles have less "sag." Don't be impatient with this exercise. It works eventually. It can actually be done anywhere, but it's easier to remember to do it if you're already exercising.

Jack-in-the-Box Squat

1. Push swing.
2. Squat down, keeping back straight, hands on knees for balance (A).
3. Jump up to starting position to meet returning swing. Push swing again.
4. Repeat five times.

Target: thighs and legs

Comment: In the beginning, you may lose your balance as you try to squat. If the exercise is difficult for you, start by squatting only halfway down. With practice, you will be able to push and squat in perfect rhythm with the swing. This exercise is also aimed at improving your balance and coordination.

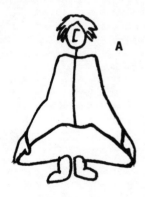

Swing Squat

1. Push swing.
2. Squat down and *remain down*, pushing returning swing five times from squatting position. If necessary, place one hand on the ground to steady yourself in the squatting position in the intervals between pushing the swing.
3. Stand up, push swing, and S-T-R-E-T-C-H.
4. Push swing and squat down. Push five more times from squatting position and then stretch once.

Target: lower back, thighs, and balance

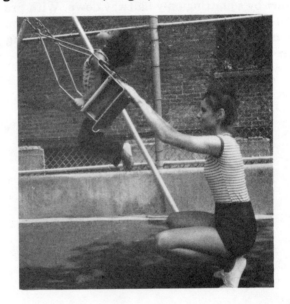

Jogging

1. Push swing.
2. Begin jogging.

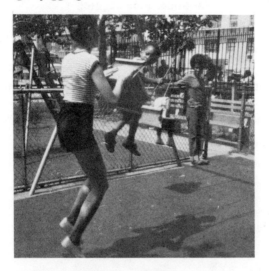

3. Without breaking your jogging rhythm, push the swing each time it returns.
4. Do fifty jogging steps, counting one step each time right foot touches ground.

Target: cardiovascular conditioning

Comment: This exercise is very simple, a good weight reducer, and a good stamina builder. If you haven't been exercising in a long time, you can probably do only about thirty jogging steps before feeling completely exhausted. That's enough for the first time. With practice, you will be able to jog for longer and longer periods of time. Jogging is a basic activity for conditioning the cardiovascular system, and fitness experts recommend that you stay at it until you feel your pulse racing for a few minutes. Many people believe that jogging is the most complete exercise there is for a total feeling of well-being.

Variation: Side Jogging

You can vary your routine of ordinary jogging by doing a side jog, as follows:

1. Jump on left foot, throwing right foot sideways (A).
2. Jump on right foot, throwing left foot sideways (B).

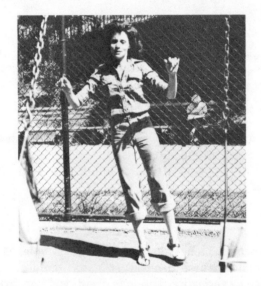

3. Establish rhythm of side jog by doing it a few times.
4. Without breaking rhythm of side jogging, push swing each time it returns.
5. Do fifty jogging steps, counting one step each time right foot touches ground.

Target: cardiovascular conditioning

Comment: Comments on jogging also apply to side jogging.

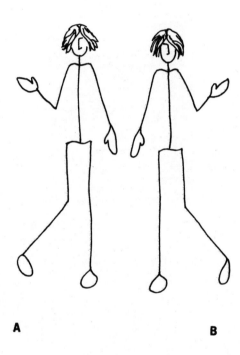

A   B

Complete Stretch

1. Stand in front of swing facing child. Grasp swing and walk backwards a few steps, holding on to swing (A).

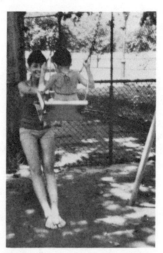

A

2. Push swing but do not let go; follow through with body (B). Feel complete S-T-R-E-T-C-H of body.

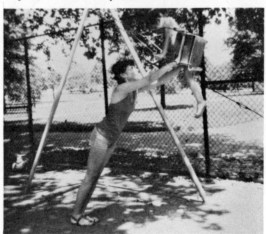

B

3. Hold for a count of five.
4. Return to position A, pulling swing with you.
5. Repeat twice.

Target: loosening up and stretching of all muscles
and joints

Comment: This exercise involves holding on to the
swing all the time and following the movement of the
swing with the natural movement of your body. Parent
and child face each other all the time. Generally, children
are delighted with this unexpected variation of the usual
swinging. They particularly like the holding action of
position B and may want you to hold it for a longer period
of time than your count of five. Do so if you can. It's a
good stretching movement for the whole body.

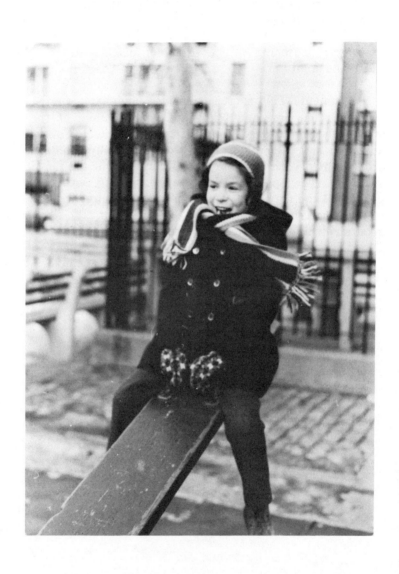

Chapter 6

One, Two, Three for the Seesaw

A young child playing on a seesaw learns that two children of approximately the same weight can manipulate the seesaw board very nicely. The child may also discover that two people of unequal weight can seesaw if the heavier person sits closer to the center than the lighter one. The lever principle that governs the operation of the seesaw has been known for hundreds of years. One may even theorize that early man discovered the lever long, long ago. We can imagine the scene: two logs, one placed over the other at a right angle, and the cave children happily popping up and down on their rudimentary seesaw. The seesaw should pose few difficulties for the twentieth-century adult. Our reactions are instinctive, and we know kinesthetically—in our muscles—how to shift our weight and position on the board to achieve a balance. However, knowledge of the lever principle may help us in manipulating the seesaw as a vehicle for exercise.

A few of the exercises in this chapter are obvious variations of exercises done with other equipment, but most are designed specifically for the seesaw. You can do a number of the exercises while helping your child use the equipment. These exercises may also be done with another adult, although in that case the balance points and leverage would be different.

We will also describe a whole series of exercises that an adult can do alone, using the seesaw as a slantboard.

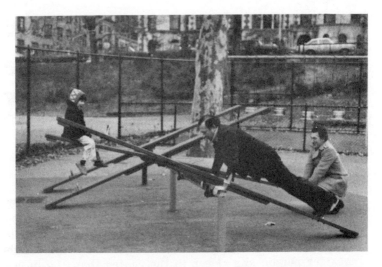

What is a slantboard? Simply a tilted board on which one exercises in a variety of positions. Instead of lying horizontally on the floor, one lies at a slant on the tilted board which intensifies the exercise process. Also, instead of carrying a mat to the park and searching for a flat area, without stones and pebbles, you have a ready-made surface on which to lie and exercise.

Not all seesaws are built to the same dimensions. Some exercises will work with your seesaw; some will not. They are designed for a standard sized board. Work slowly and cautiously to find those exercises you can use and then proceed more vigorously. When you have learned the basic uses of the seesaw, you can probably improvise on your own. For example, you may be able to adapt your favorite exercises for use on the seesaw, modifying or intensifying them as you see fit.

We remind you again that any of the calisthenic-type exercises, such as the Seesaw Sit-up or the Seesaw Push-up, if performed with sufficient intensity and duration, can serve as a conditioning activity that has a beneficial effect on the cardiovascular system.

Seesaw Pump

1. With your child seated at one end of seesaw, stand at other end, feet together, hands on board in front of you (A, page 68).
2. Press slowly down on board with both hands, keeping legs straight, until board touches ground (B).

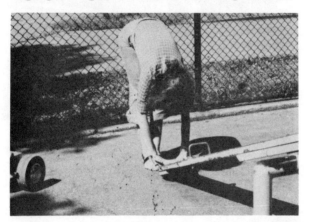

3. Hold in down position for a count of ten, feeling S-T-R-E-T-C-H in spine. Be sure that knees are *not* bent.
4. Release slowly, keeping board under control as it slowly goes up (and your child, at other end, slowly goes down).
5. Repeat five times.

Target: thighs and back

Comment: This is the most obvious exercise for the seesaw. It is the most usual way of pumping the seesaw and most adults do it this way. You can vary this exercise by starting with your legs two feet apart. This wider stance results in increased stretching of the legs and upper thighs.

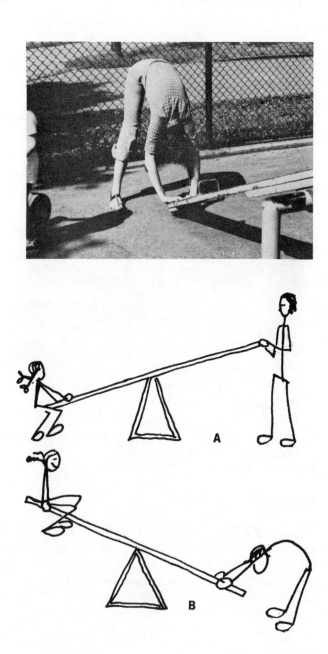

Seesaw Squat

1. Stand erect, feet together, at one end of seesaw. (Your child is seated on board at other end.) Place hands on board.
2. Press down on board, simultaneously lowering trunk, and bending knees until you are squatting on your heels.

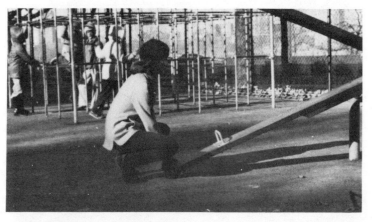

3. Hold for count of five.
4. Rise gradually to erect position as your child slowly descends.
5. Repeat five times.

Target: arms, legs, and thighs

Comment: If you can't go all the way down, go as far as you can and then push the board to ground level by leaning forward (so that your child has his turn to be high in the air). This exercise is like the classic calisthenic knee bend except that you can steady yourself by grasping the seesaw board. As a result, you should be able to go lower than you otherwise could and eventually you should be able to sit back on your heels.

Seesaw Back Kick

1. Stand about one foot from one end of seesaw, facing your child who is sitting on other end. Place hands on board (A).
2. Press board down to ground, simultaneously raising left leg high into air (B).
3. Hold for count of five. Feel S-T-R-E-T-C-H.
4. Gradually return to standing position, keeping board under control as your child's end of board slowly descends.
5. Repeat, this time raising right leg.

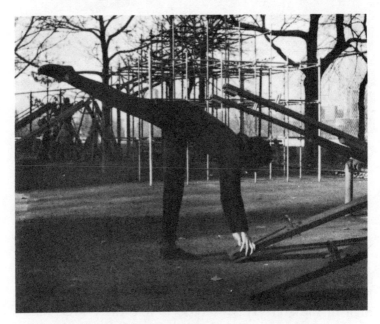

6. Repeat exercise, alternating legs, until you have raised each leg five times.

Target: arms and legs

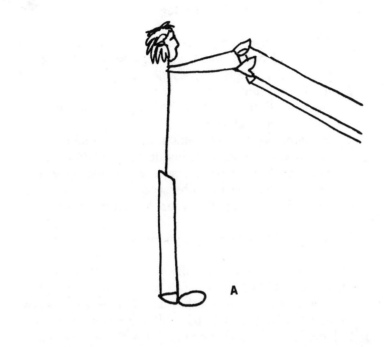

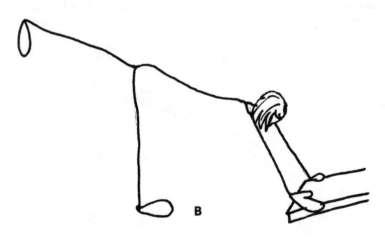

Seesaw Jog

1. Stand at raised end of seesaw; place both hands on end of board and begin jogging. As you jog, raise feet as high as possible (A).
2. Jog for a count of ten.
3. Push board down and let it rise gradually during another count of ten.
4. Do three such sets (which means a count of sixty and which also means up-down-up-down-up-down for your end of the seesaw and the reverse for your child on the other end.)
5. Relax. Repeat only if you are not too tired.

Target: cardiovascular conditioning

Comment: It is worthwhile to work out a jogging rhythm with each of the various apparatus in the playground. You may find another rhythm at the seesaw which better suits you and your child. If you only manage to do jogging at the playground, you will still have made a very positive step towards physical fitness. All comments made about jogging at the swings also apply here.

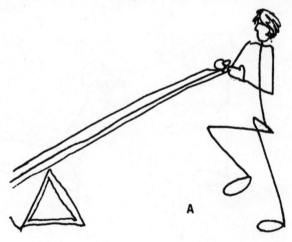

A

THE SEESAW AS SLANTBOARD

Try these only when there is an empty seesaw and your child is busy and happy elsewhere.

Seesaw Twist

1. Sit on seesaw board, feet resting on bottom handle.
2. Cross left leg over right leg, placing left foot near right knee.
3. Place left hand on seesaw board about six inches behind you, twisting trunk to do so.
4. Bring right hand over left knee, grasping right knee and turning as far as possible to left. Look in direction of left hand (A).

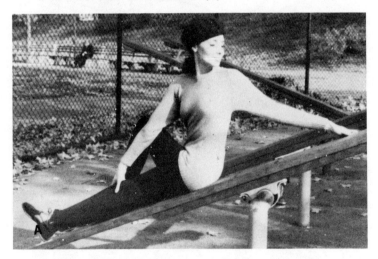

5. Feel S-T-R-E-T-C-H in waist and hold for count of ten.
6. Relax, recover, and reverse.

Target: waist

Isometric Posture Improver

1. Lie down on seesaw, head higher than feet.
2. Bend knees, resting feet on handle at lower end of board.
3. Bend arms, holding on to board in area of waistline (A). Be aware of space between middle back and board.
4. Press lumbar region against board, trying to narrow space as much as possible (B).
5. Hold for a count of ten. Relax.
6. Repeat twice.

Target: pelvic alignment

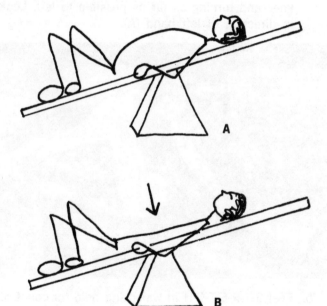

Abdominal Press

1. Lie down on seesaw, head higher than feet and feet resting on handle at lower end of board.
2. Place both hands behind head (A, page 76).
3. Raise trunk to form a forty-five-degree angle with board (B).

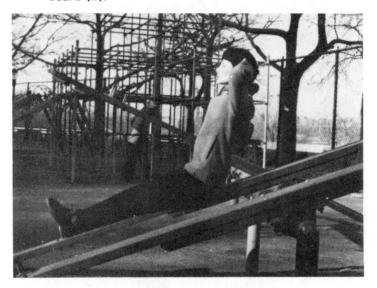

4. Contract abdomen and hold for count of five.
5. Relax.

Target: abdomen

Comment: As in all isometric exercises, the benefits are proportional to the effort put into that five second hold. If you find it too difficult to raise your trunk from the board with your hands behind your head, then try a slightly easier position: stretch your hands out in front of you for balance (C). After you have mastered this, do exercise with hands behind head.

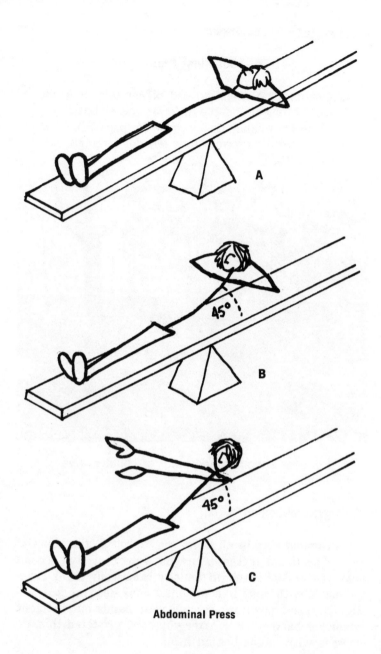

Abdominal Press

Seesaw Sit-up

1. Lie down on board, face up, head higher than feet.
2. Rest both feet on handle at lower end of board and place hands behind head (A, page 78).
3. Without moving legs, slowly sit up (B). (If this is too difficult for you, then go back to lying position and raise both arms overhead. Then slowly sit up, bringing out-stretched arms from overhead to frontal position to help gain momentum.) (C)

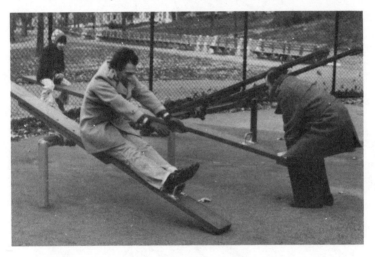

4. With hands behind head, slowly return to lying position.
5. Do five sit-ups.

Target: abdomen and upper thighs

Comment: To vary this routine, do the following. In the sitting position (step 3), reach out and try to touch your toes. Hold this for a five-second stretch. This added movement can easily be worked into the rhythm and routine of this exercise.

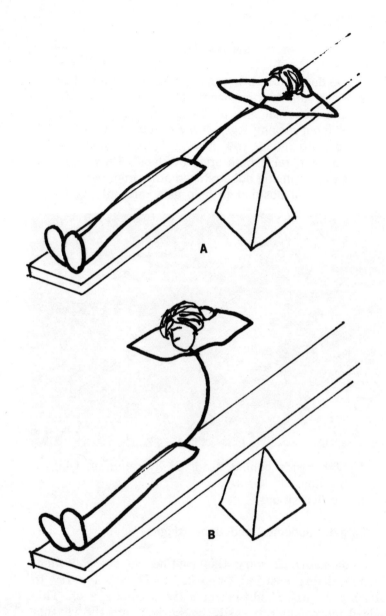

Seesaw Sit-up

Touch Toe Sit-up

1. Lie down on board, face up, head higher than feet, arms stretched overhead.
2. Raise trunk and right leg from board to form a V position (A).

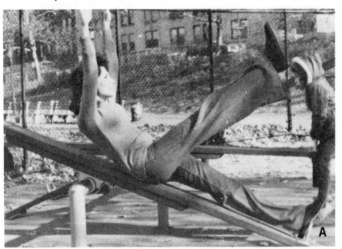

3. Touch left hand to right toes and hold for a count of five (B).

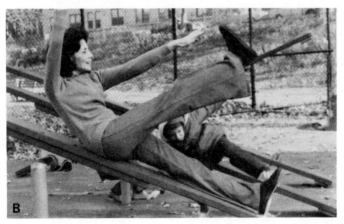

4. Return to supine position.
5. Repeat, this time raising left leg from board and touching left toes with right hand. Hold for count of five.
6. Return to supine position.
7. Repeat five times.

Target: abdomen, arms, shoulders, and spine

Back Stretch

1. Lie down on board, face up, head higher than feet.
2. Rest both feet on handle at lower end of board and raise arms overhead.
3. Slowly raise trunk to sitting position (A, page 82).
4. Place hands on knees and slowly bend forward, flexing arms (B). (Aim forehead toward knees.)

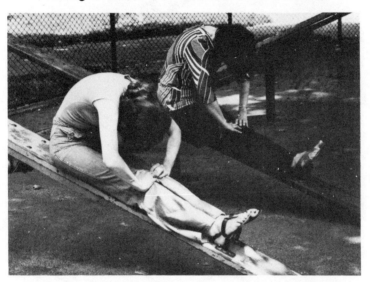

5. Hold for count of ten. Feel S-T-R-E-T-C-H in spine.
6. Relax.

Target. a more flexible spine

Comment: This exercise is aimed at giving you a slow, easy stretch in the lumbar area. If you find it easy to do, then try the same exercise grasping calves of legs instead of knees. When you have mastered this second position, go on to the most difficult position: bending forwards to grasp ankles. The yogis have the expression,

"You are as young as your spine is flexible."[1] This exercise is aimed at giving you a more flexible spine.

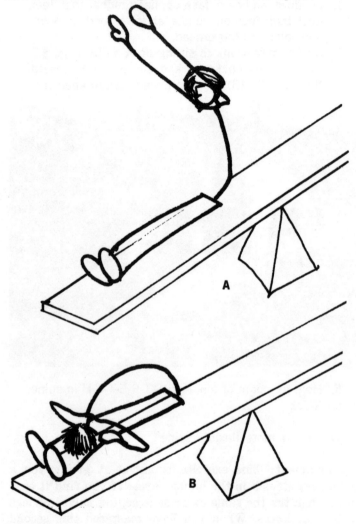

A

B

1. Richard Hittleman, *Yoga 28 Day Exercise Plan* (New York: Workman, 1969), p. 19.

Serpent

1. Lie face down on board, feet lower than head, forehead pressing against board.
2. Rest feet on lower handle.
3. Place hands on board beneath shoulders, elbows bent.
4. Keeping hips in contact with board, tilt head backward and raise upper trunk from board, partially unbending elbows.

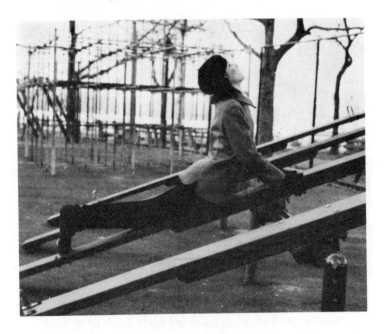

5. Feel S-T-R-E-T-C-H in curved spine.
6. Hold for count of ten.
7. Slowly lower trunk back to board and relax.
8. Repeat three times.

Target: lower back

Seesaw Push-up

1. Lie face down on board with head higher than feet.
2. Rest feet on lower handle.
3. Grasp crossbar (structural bar on which seesaw board rests) with both hands, palms down, elbows bent.
4. Straighten elbows, keeping body stiff and lifting trunk and upper thighs from board.

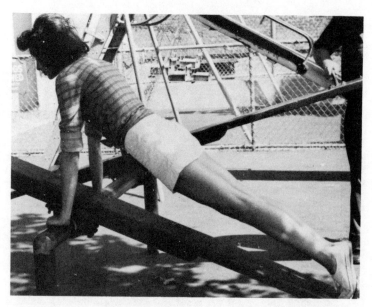

5. Slowly bend elbows, lowering body back to board.
6. Do five push-ups.

Target: upper arms, shoulders, and abdomen

Seesaw Cat

1. Lie face down on board, head higher than feet.
2. Rest feet on lower handle.
3. Grasp sides of board with both hands, palms down, elbows bent.
4. Tuck head down, chin against chest, and push away from board. Bend knees and straighten elbows as you glide hands down board.
5. Sit back on heels in "cat" position. Hold for count of ten. Feel S-T-R-E-T-C-H in spine.
6. Return to original position.
7. Repeat three times.

Target: upper arms, shoulders, and spine

Comment: This exercise can be worked into a continuous routine with the previous exercise, the Seesaw Push-Up. Begin with a push-up, pushing away from the board instead of the crossbar, and then continue into "cat" position.

Side Lift

1. Lie down on seesaw on your left side, head higher than feet, left foot resting against lower handle.
2. Raise head and support it with your left hand, left elbow on board. With right hand, grasp side of board for support and balance (A).
3. Slowly raise right leg as high as possible (B).
4. Feel S-T-R-E-T-C-H in right leg and hold for count of five.
5. Slowly bring right leg down; relax.
6. Turn over to right side and perform mirror image of steps 1–5.

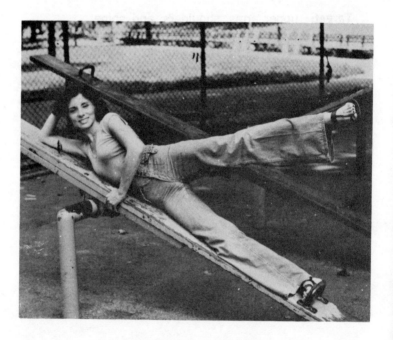

Target: abdomen, hips, and thighs

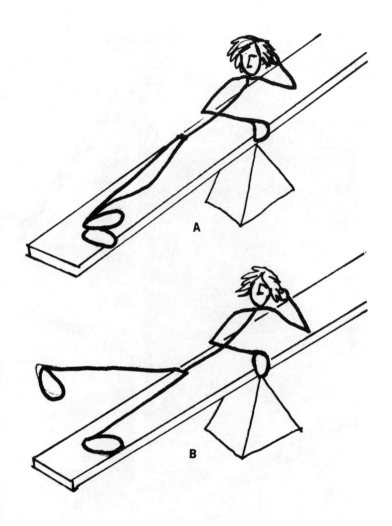

A

B

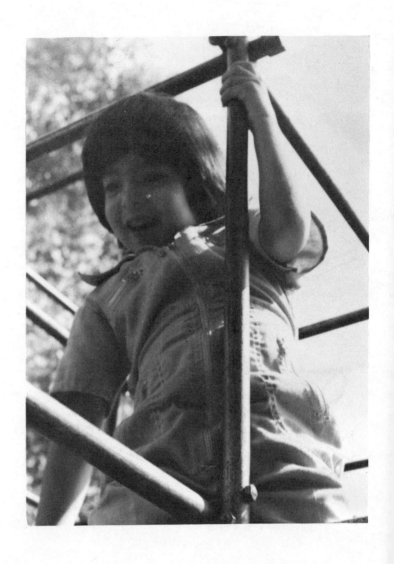

Chapter 7

Jungle
Gymnastics

The jungle gym brings to mind images of apes swinging on vines in the jungle, of Tarzan swinging from tree to tree as he goes to rescue his Jane. It evokes some atavistic instinct in all of us to hang by the hands, swing in the air, and use this swinging motion as a form of locomotion. No, you say? Well, think of how a newborn baby will grasp an offered finger. Experiments have shown that an infant will clasp a bar firmly enough to hang by his hands for a few seconds. This clasping response, known as the Moro reflex, is something basic to every human being, probably coming from the past of the human race itself. This response, long forgotten, can be relearned. Children do it with ease.

The jungle gym is a versatile structure that invites climbing, hanging by the hands, sitting upright, or hanging upside down. Most children who haven't been inhibited by taboos and cautions and "Don't do this" and "Don't do that" love to climb higher and higher on this piece of equipment and survey the world from the top. It's a place to get rid of feelings of smallness and inferiority and to test oneself and one's agility over and over again.

The jungle gym has fallen into disrepute lately, as has other classic playground equipment. Somehow, the innovators in playground design feel that free-form

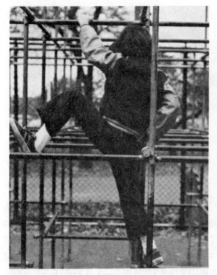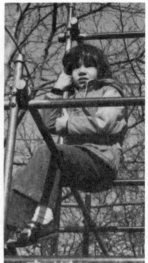

equipment, not so traditional in design, is more stimulating to children and less boring.

Actually, it is only the adults who are bored. The equipment, old to us, is new to every child when he first discovers it. If we could look at this apparatus with the fresh eyes of childhood, we might see it quite differently.

Most jungle gyms are simply constructed and rigidly geometric in form; yet the apparatus allows for more innovation in activity and movement than any other piece of equipment in the park. In a way, it's like sand: it's exactly what you make of it. Our question is, What can we, as adults, make of it?

We don't suggest climbing the jungle gym to get to the top. We don't know whether it's constructed to hold up under the weight of adults. It's really not necessary, for our purposes, to try it. As climbing apparatus, it should be reserved for children. (Let this be one place where they can really look down on grownups.)

At the jungle gym, the parent is usually not directly involved with the child's play (as he is at the swings or

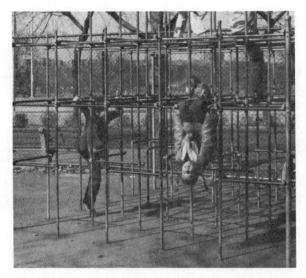

seesaw, pushing or pumping to help the child function on the equipment). Of course, from time to time, the child may seek help in doing what he wants to do and is too timid to try, but a parent's role here is limited. However, when the parent exercises at the jungle gym while the child climbs, the two of them have a true parallel play situation, each doing his own thing independently but side by side.

Most young children find great pleasure in sharing a piece of equipment with a parent, even though each is using it for a different purpose. It is as if the parent says: "What we are doing is important. It's important for you, and it's also important for me." Parallel play is a serious acceptance of the child's world by action rather than by words.

It is sometimes exciting for children to feel that their playthings can have serious adult uses. One friend recently told us of an event in her childhood that made a great impression on her. The family stove was not working, and one of her toys, a miniature electric stove,

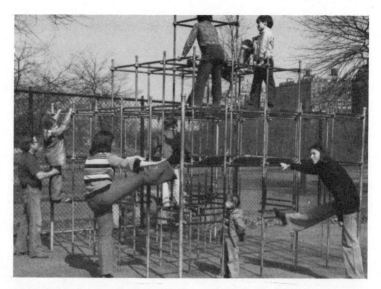

was used to heat dinner. She suddenly felt her plaything had a real function in the adult world too. Other children can feel the same way when they see the jungle gym being used by their parents for exercise.

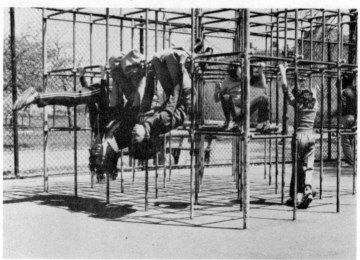

We will describe in this chapter jungle gym exercises for the parent alone. Most of them use the two lower rungs of the apparatus. One exercise, Jungle Animals, is for parent and child, and it is open ended: you can make of it what you will. Most of the exercises are to be done in a parallel situation with the child. Some may be incorporated into a variety of games that almost every parent and child know—for example, "Follow the Leader," "Simple Simon," "Monkey Sees, Monkey Does"—with parent and child alternating leadership.

The conditioning activity at the jungle gym may be either fast-paced calisthenics or jogging, and these need no further description.

The following exercises are designed for standard-sized jungle gyms found in most city parks. Be aware of any differences between your apparatus and the apparatus shown here, and modify the instructions accordingly.

Imaginary Chair

1. Stand about nine inches from corner of jungle
   gym, back to corner pole. Lean against pole, placing hands on thighs.
2. Imagine there is a chair between you and the pole
   and slowly lower your body to a sitting position.
   As you move down, your back should press against
   the pole and your hands should slide toward your
   knees (A).

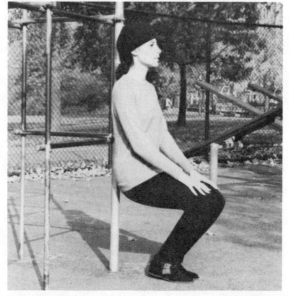

A

3. Hold for five to seven seconds in sitting position.
4. Return to starting position by sliding body slowly
   up the pole, keeping upper and lower back in contact with the pole.
5. Relax.
6. Repeat twice.

Target: upper thighs and calves

Posture Improver

1. Stand erect, back to corner pole of jungle gym.
2. Lean against pole, being aware of space between your back and the pole.
3. Contract abdomen and press lumbar area against the pole, trying to narrow the space as much as possible. Stand with your back flat against pole (A).

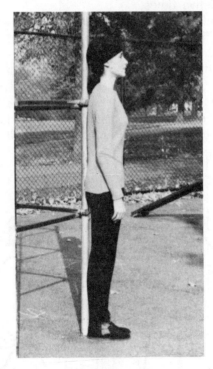

A

4. Hold for count of five to seven seconds.
5. Relax.

Target: abdomen, pelvic alignment, posture improvement

Jungle Knee Bend

1. Stand about one arm's length from jungle gym,
   right side toward apparatus.
2. Extend right arm and grasp lowest rung of apparatus; place left hand on hip (A).
3. Keeping body erect, bend knees and lower trunk until sitting on heels (heels off ground) (B).
4. Stand up again, keeping body erect.
5. Repeat five times.
6. Turn left side toward jungle gym and repeat exercise five times.

Target: thighs and calves

Comment: If you can't reach a full knee bend, then start with a quarter knee bend; over a period of time, proceed to a half knee bend and then to a full knee bend.

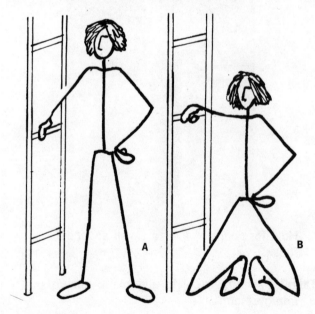

Jungle Push-up

1. Stand one body length from jungle gym, facing apparatus.
2. Bend over and grasp bottom bar with both hands, palms down.
3. Flex elbows and lower body as close as you can to bottom bar. Keep body as stiff as possible.

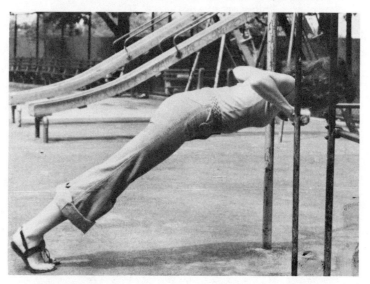

4. Straighten arms and push body an arm's length up from bar.
5. Repeat five times.
6. Relax.

Target: upper arms and shoulders

Comment: As you become more skilled in this exercise you will be able to touch your chest to the lower bar. Don't worry if you can't do it right away, and don't force it. In time, you will master this exercise.

Jungle Stretch

1. Stand facing jungle gym about one foot away, feet together. Grasp rung nearest shoulder level with both hands, palms down (A, page 100).
2. Lean backward, stretching arms, curving spine, and "sagging" towards ground. Feel as if jungle gym is moving at full speed and you are holding on and "blowing in the wind" (B).

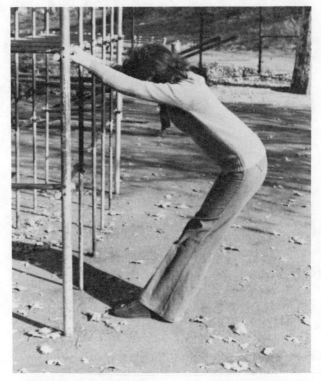

3. Hold for count of three. Feel S-T-R-E-T-C-H in spine and upper arms.
4. Stand up straight, rise on toes, tilt head backward, and arch spine (C).

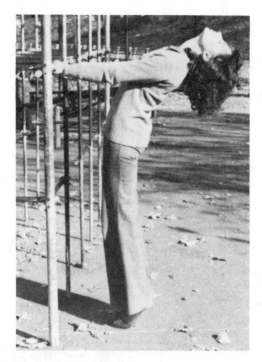

5. Hold for count of three.
6. Alternate positions, each time holding **extreme** position for count of three.
7. Repeat five times.

Target: arms, legs, and spine

Comment: On rainy days, you can easily do this exercise at home. Instead of holding on to the jungle gym, you can grasp the two handles of an open door.

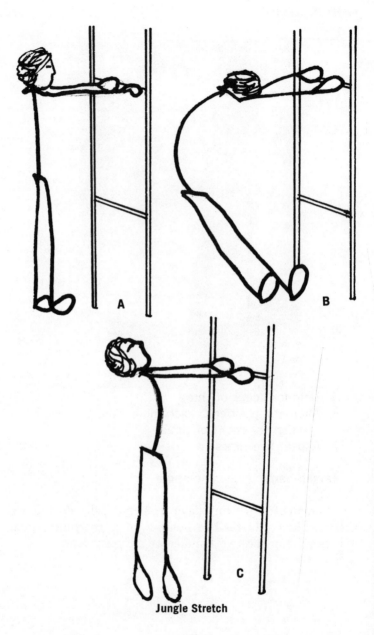

Jungle Stretch

Leg Stretch

1. Place left foot on first rung of jungle gym.
2. Raise both arms above head.
3. Bend forward, grasping leg at calf (A).

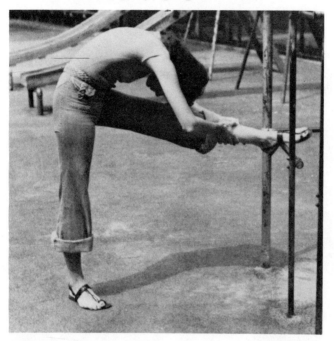

A

4. Flex elbows, bringing trunk closer to left leg and feeling S-T-R-E-T-C-H in spine.
5. Hold for count of five.
6. Relax.
7. Repeat, this time placing right foot on first rung of jungle gym and going through steps 1–6.

Target: thighs and flexible spine

Comment: As you become more skillful in this exercise, grasp the ankle instead of the calf in step 3.

Jungle Arch

1. Stand facing jungle gym at place where there is no bottom rung.
2. Grasp bar in second row with both hands, palms down.
3. Place right foot on bottom bar of inner jungle gym.
4. Shift weight to right foot and place left foot alongside right foot on bottom bar.
5. Supported by hands and feet, tilt head backward and arch spine. (A)

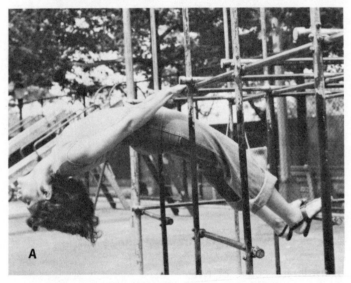

A

6. Feel S-T-R-E-T-C-H in spine and hold for count of ten.
7. Return to original position by straightening back and stepping down from bar.
8. Relax.

Target: spine, neck, arms, and legs

Jungle Lunge

1. Stand about arm's length from jungle gym, facing apparatus.
2. Extend right arm and grasp rung nearest shoulder level.
3. Bend left leg behind you and grasp left foot with left hand, tilting body forward (A, page 104).
4. Feel S-T-R-E-T-C-H in left leg and arm.
5. Hold for count of five.
6. Relax.
7. Repeat, this time extending left arm to grasp nearest rung and grasping right leg with right hand. (B)

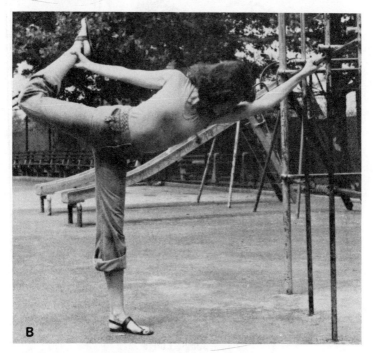

B

Target: thighs, arms, and shoulders

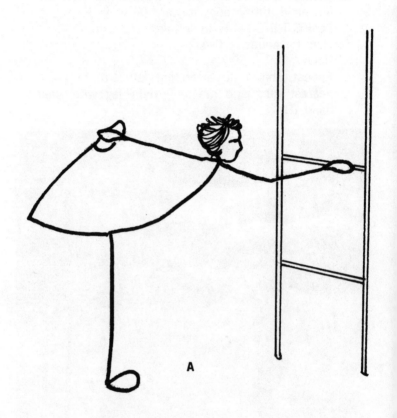

A

Jungle Lunge

Jungle Squeeze

1. Sit on bottom rung of jungle gym; tilt slightly backward so that head is behind second rung.
2. Place hands on vertical bars on both sides of hips, just above bottom rung, palms forward (A).
3. Keep body stiff and press sideways with hands, holding for count of five to seven seconds.
4. Relax. Place hands at shoulder level on same bars, palms forward (B, page 106).
5. Press sideways again, holding for count of five to seven seconds.
6. Relax. Place hands on same bars as high as you can reach. Elbows should be straight (C).
7. Press sideways for five to seven seconds.
8. Relax.

Target: chest and upper arms

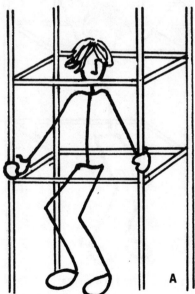

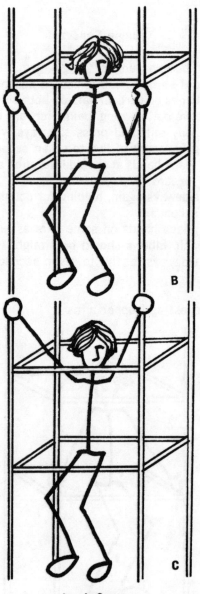

Jungle Squeeze

Jungle Kick

1. Stand about one arm's length from jungle gym, right side toward apparatus.
2. Extend right arm and grasp rung nearest shoulder level.
3. Extend left arm sideways and parallel to ground. Raise left leg as high as possible toward left hand.
4. Hold for count of five and feel S-T-R-E-T-C-H.
5. Relax.
6. About face, and repeat the same procedure in mirror image of steps 1–5.

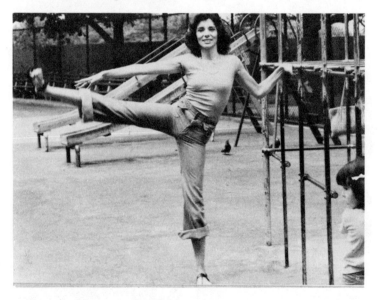

Target: legs and thighs

Comment: This exercise is like a long, slow kick, holding and stretching at the peak. It's not at all necessary to actually touch foot to hand; the benefits are derived from the process of holding and stretching.

Dangling in the Jungle

1. Stand facing jungle gym at place where there is
   no bottom rung.
2. Grasp rung at second level, palms down.
3. Place feet on bottom rung in inner jungle gym (A).

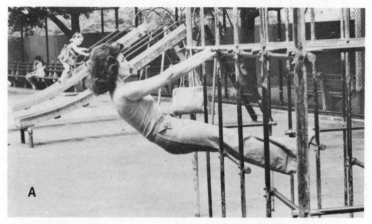

4. Flex knees, keeping weight of body on right leg.
   Carefully bring left leg up over bar that hands
   are grasping (B).

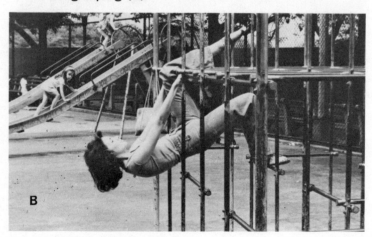

5. Shift weight to left leg and hook right knee over bar between left leg and right hand (C).

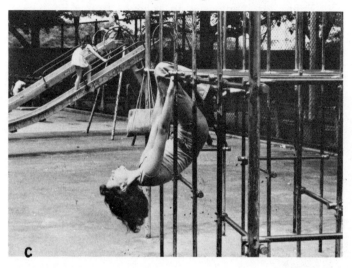

C

6. Dangle by legs, placing hands on ground for additional support if necessary (D).

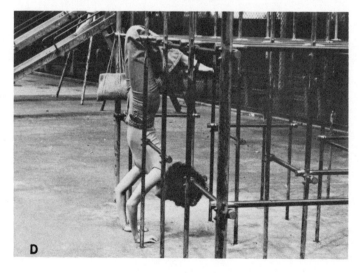

D

7. Hold for count of ten. Feel complete S-T-R-E-T-C-H of legs and spine.
8. There are two ways to recover from this position. One way is to go directly into the Jungle Somersault (next page). The other way is simply to go back the way you came—that is, grasp the same bar that supports your legs (C); place right leg on inner bottom rung (B); bring left leg to rest on same rung (A); return both feet to ground; and release hold on second rung.

Target: upper thighs, spine, and stimulation of cardiovascular system

Comment: This is an upside-down position. The yogis attach great importance to such positions because they believe a person benefits when the blood rushes to the head. You can judge for yourself.

Jungle Somersault

1. Go through steps 1–5 of Dangling in the Jungle so that you arrive at position C of that exercise.
2. Remove hands from second rung and grasp vertical bars on each side of you.
3. Remove legs from rung and carefully bring them forward, hanging by your hands (A).
4. Propel yourself around, feet towards ground and head away from ground; land with feet on ground.

Target: upper arms, increased agility

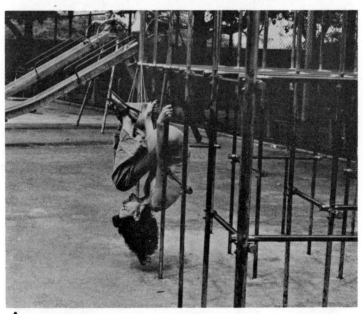

A

Jungle Animals

1. Stand erect, facing jungle gym.
2. Lean forward placing hands on upper thighs and looking through bars of jungle gym.
3. Slowly extend and stretch fingers.
4. Simultaneously open your eyes as wide as possible, stick out your tongue as far as possible, and feel like a ferocious jungle animal—lion, tiger, or what have you (A).

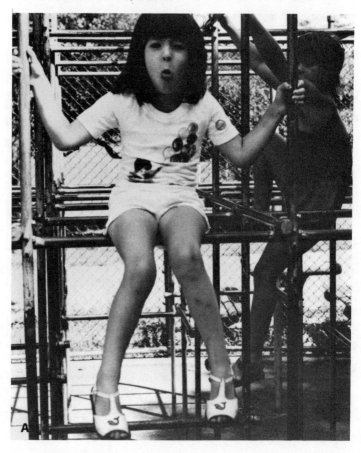

5. Hold for count of ten.
6. Repeat twice.

Target: face and neck muscles

Comment: This is an exercise traditionally associated with yoga. Yogis call it "The Lion" and do it sitting on the floor. We feel it is suitable for the jungle gym. In fact, the exercise can serve as a springboard for a whole series of exercises. You can growl while doing it if it helps increase the pleasure and fun for children. You and your children might find this an opportunity for innovation and develop a series of animal exercises that incorporate foot and body movements as well as facial expressions and grimaces. You might consider the following exercises and then go on to create your own:

1. Flapping wings (arms) and flying (leaping) to imitate eagles, sea gulls, pigeons, or other birds.
2. Running, punctuated every few steps with a jump, to imitate the movements of squirrels.
3. Walking heavily, hands clasped with arms straight and swinging and body turning from side to side to imitate the characteristic movements of an elephant.
4. Alternate jumping and squatting to imitate rabbits.
5. A waddling walk to imitate ducks.
6. Cantering or galloping to imitate horses.

You take it from here!

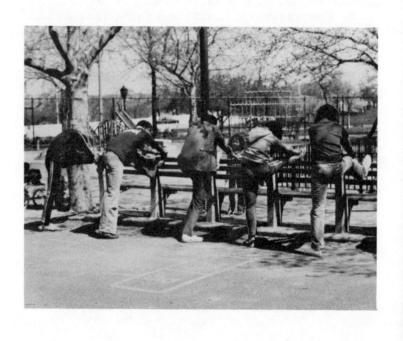

Chapter 8

Back
to the Bench

This chapter presents a series of exercises using the park bench itself as the primary apparatus, and also aerobic activities using the general park area near the bench as the field of exercise. You may turn to these exercises and activities when other park equipment has been preempted or when you find yourself working alone because your child is busy elsewhere. Some of you may feel less conspicuous exercising at the bench and, in fact, may prefer it even though other pieces of equipment are available. The aerobic activity in the bench area may be either regular jogging—which can be done close to the bench or circling the playground area—or rope jumping, which we regard as an ideal playground activity for parents and children.

Park bench exercises meet several special needs. They can be used by anyone who wants to exercise in the park. They lend themselves easily to group work since, in most parks, benches are in plentiful supply and there is consequently no problem of finding enough available equipment. Finally, the park bench exercises can easily be used with a chair at home on cold or rainy days when parent and child are indoors and the parent does not want to miss an exercise day.

So here we go, back to the bench.

Bench Push-up

1. Stand a few feet behind bench, feet flat on ground, body straight. Lean forward and grasp back of bench, arms parallel and straight.
2. Slowly bend elbows and lower chest toward bench, body straight as a board. Rise on toes at same time.

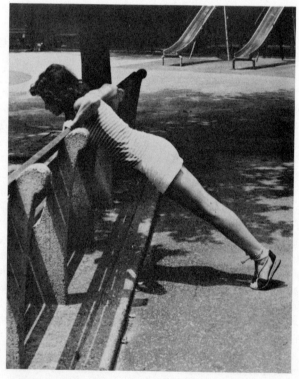

3. Straighten arms and push yourself back to upright posture.
4. Repeat five times.

Target: upper arms and shoulders

Bench Lift

1. Stand right side next to front of bench. Extend arms sideways at shoulder level for balance (A, page 118).
2. Place right foot on bench (B).
3. Slowly shift weight to right leg, simultaneously raising left foot to bench level (C). Feel tension in your right leg as you do this. If you feel no tension you're doing it too quickly: slow down.
4. Stand with both feet on bench (D).
5. Slowly extend left leg to side and gradually lower it to ground. Shift weight to left leg and bring right foot down to ground (A).

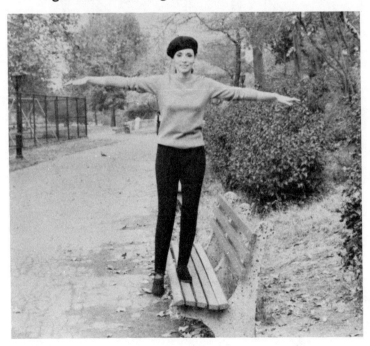

6. About face and do mirror image of steps 1–5.
7. Do two complete bench lifts.

Target: thighs and legs

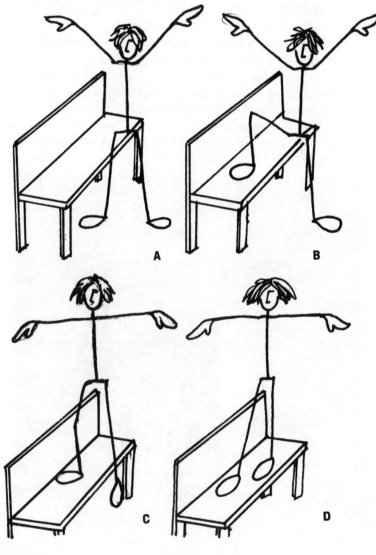

Back Bench Stretch

1. Stand back to back with bench, approximately one foot away from it.
2. Grasp top of bench with both hands (A).
3. Holding on to bench, walk away as far as you can. Rise on toes. Tilt head backward, arch spine, and S-T-R-E-T-C-H (B). Press down on bench.

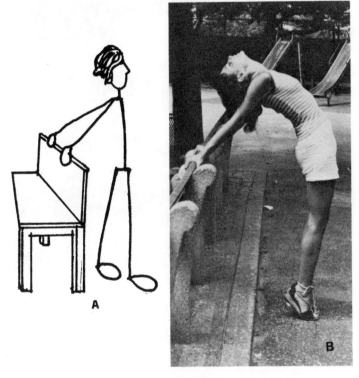

4. Hold this position for a count of five.
5. Move back to original position and relax.
6. Repeat twice.

Target: back, arms, and thighs

Inverted Back Bench Stretch

1. Begin as in Back Bench Stretch and follow through to position B. (See previous page.)
2. Still holding on to bench, relax arched back, tilt head forward, contract abdomen and let body sink toward ground, position A, this page.

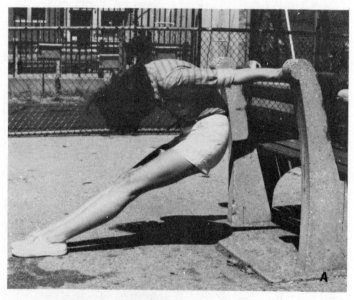

3. Hold for a count of five.
4. Pushing with both hands, move back to arched position B.
5. Return to original position and relax.
6. Repeat twice.

Target: arms, neck, and abdomen

Isometric Ankle Twist

1. Sit erect on bench, hands gripping edge of bench.
2. Cross right ankle over left ankle.
3. Press ankles against each other.
4. Hold with maximum pressure, ankle against ankle, for count of five to seven seconds.
5. Relax; repeat exercise with ankles in reversed position.

Target: calves, legs, and thighs

Isometric Neck Twist

1. Sit on bench and turn head to right.
2. Cradle chin in palm of right hand; cover top of head with palm of left hand.
3. Simultaneously press left hand down and press right hand up while tilting head upward.

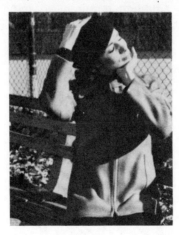

4. Hold for five to seven seconds.
5. Relax. Repeat exercise with head turned to left and hands in reversed position.

Target: neck muscles

Comment: If you have a pinched nerve in the neck region, a "pain in the neck," this is a good exercise for relieving pressure on the pinched nerve.

Isometric Bench Lift

1. Sit erect on bench, hands grasping front edge of bench (A).
2. Tense muscles of arms as if you were trying to lift bench from ground with yourself seated on it. Of course this can't be done, but that's the immovable situation required in isometrics.
3. Hold intense effort for five to seven seconds.
4. Relax.

Target: shoulders and upper arms

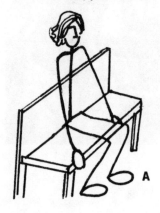

Isometric Abdominal Squeeze

1. Sit erect on bench.
2. Raise legs, extending them out straight ahead of you; also extend arms out straight ahead of you (A).

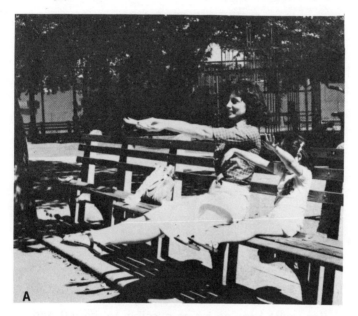

A

3. In this position, contract muscles of abdomen intensely, pushing your back against back of bench.
4. Hold for five to seven seconds.
5. Relax.

Target: abdomen

Elbow Twist

1. Sit erect on bench. Place both hands behind head (A).
2. Bend forward and turn slightly to left so that right elbow touches right knee (B). In this posi-

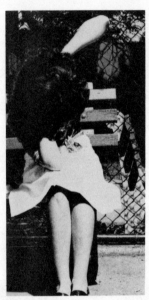

   tion, twist body as far as possible to the left and hold for a count of five, feeling S-T-R-E-T-C-H in waist.
3. Recover and bend forward again, this time turning slightly to right so that left elbow touches left knee (C). In this position, twist body as far as possible to right and hold for count of five, again feeling S-T-R-E-T-C-H in waist.
4. Repeat sequence three times.
5. Bend forward and turn more sharply to left so that right elbow touches left knee. Hold for a count of five.

6. Recover and bend forward again, turning more sharply to right so that left elbow touches right knee. Hold for a count of five.
7. Repeat steps 5 and 6 three times.
8. Relax.

Target: waist

Comment: This exercise is aimed at trimming and slimming the waist. Steps 5, 6, and 7 represent the more advanced procedures and should be tried only when steps 1 through 4 are easily done.

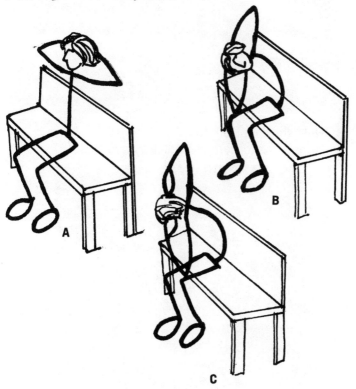

Bench Balance

1. Lie down on bench, face up.
2. Grasp sides of bench and raise trunk and legs from bench so that they form ninety-degree angle (A).

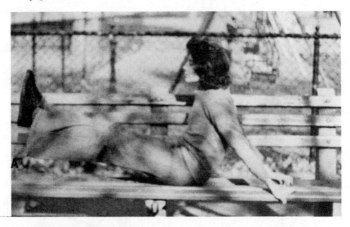

3. Hold for count of five.
4. Bring arms forward and reach toward toes. (B)

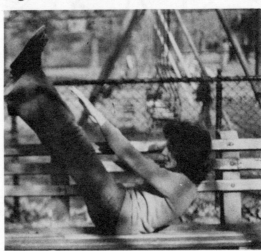

5. Relax.
6. Repeat three times.

Target: abdomen, balance, and coordination

Comment: If it is too difficult to attain the V position in step 2, then start by raising legs only a few inches from bench. With practice, eventually you will be able to attain the V position shown in (A).

Backward Bend

1. Straddle the bench, sitting erect. If your bench is a type that can't be straddled in the middle, try the end.
2. Place your hands on the bench behind you and "walk" the palms of your hands to a position twelve to fourteen inches away from your back (A).
3. Arch back and simultaneously tilt head backward, seeing the world upside down (B).

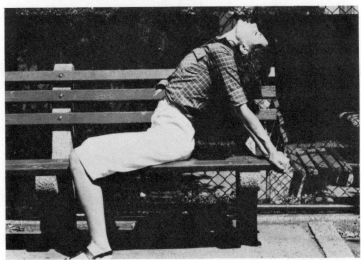

4. Hold for count of ten. Feel S-T-R-E-T-C-H in arched back.
5. Relax.

Target: back and neck muscles

Comment: After practice makes this exercise easy, try it with the palms of your hands (in step 2) about 18 inches from your back. This position results in a more intensive stretch.

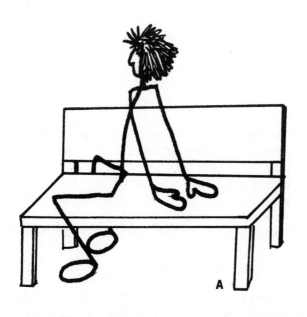

A

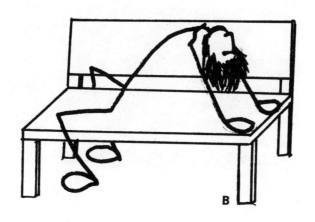

B

Bench Knee Bend

1. Stand one arm's length from back of bench, right side nearest bench.
2. Grasp top of bench with right hand. Place left hand on hip.
3. Keeping body erect, bend knees and lower trunk until sitting on your heels. Heels should be off ground.
4. Straighten knees and stand up, keeping body erect.
5. Repeat five times.
6. About face; do mirror image of steps 1–5.

Target: legs and balance

Comment: If you can't reach a full knee bend, start with a quarter knee bend and gradually increase depth of bend. After achieving the full knee bend begin practicing it with both hands on hips (without the support of the bench).

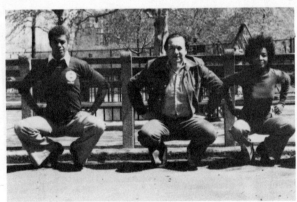

Bench Kick

1. Stand one arm's length from back of bench, left side nearest bench.
2. Grasp top of bench with left hand (A).
3. Extend right arm sideways and parallel to ground. Lift your right leg as high as you can, aiming at your right hand (B).
4. Hold for count of five and feel S-T-R-E-T-C-H.
5. Relax.
6. About face; do mirror image of steps 1–5.

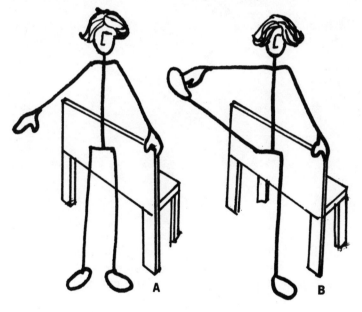

Target: legs and thighs

Comments: This exercise is like the Jungle Kick, holding and stretching at the peak. You probably won't be able to touch foot to hand. It doesn't matter. The benefits are derived from the stretching and holding.

Bench Lunge

1. Stand facing back of bench about half a body
   length away.
2. Extend right arm and grasp top of bench with right
   hand.
3. Bend left leg behind you and grasp left ankle
   with left hand.
4. Tilt body forward (A).

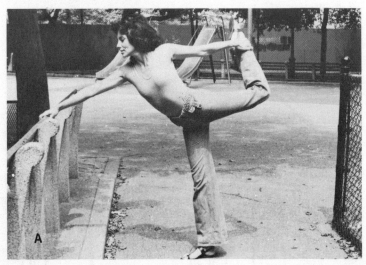

5. Hold for count of five and feel S-T-R-E-T-C-H.
6. Slowly return to original position. Relax.
7. Repeat steps 1–6, reversing left-right positions.

Target: thighs and balance

Comment: As you become more proficient in this
exercise, you may want to try a more advanced version
of it. Do the exercise without the support of the bench
back. Simply extend one arm in front of you to help to
keep your balance.

Spinal Stretch

1. Stand facing back of bench, one arm's length from it.
2. Extend right leg; rest it on top of bench back.
3. Extend both arms above head and slowly bend forward. Grasp right knee in both hands and bend elbows to bring chest closer to knee.
4. Hold for count of ten, feeling S-T-R-E-T-C-H in back and upper right thigh.
5. Assume original position and relax.
6. Repeat steps 2–4 with left leg extended.
7. Relax.

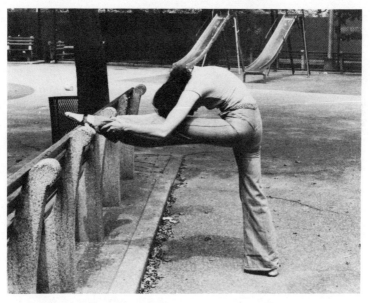

Target: spine and thighs

Comment: As you develop skill in this exercise you will be able to grasp the calf and, eventually, the ankle. Such agility comes with a more flexible spine, which is one goal of this stretching exercise. To gain flexibility does take practice, and improvement comes inch by inch; so don't be discouraged. You will probably notice some improvement each time you practice.

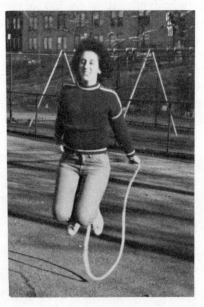

AEROBIC ACTIVITIES

In looking for aerobic activities suitable for the bench area, we turn naturally to jogging and rope jumping.

Either activity should be done long enough and intensely enough to achieve a conditioning effect. We remind you that it is generally believed that an activity must increase the pulse rate for at least a minute or two in order to train the cardiovascular and respiratory systems. It would be advisable to check with your own physician to see what pulse rate schedule is suitable for you.

Many exercise theorists recommend a jogging schedule of fifty jogging steps alternating with ten walking steps, hops, or jumps. A beginner should do only one set the first day and gradually increase the amount of activity, judging for himself how far and how fast to go.

Since we have already discussed jogging in several other chapters, we will focus here in greater detail on rope jumping as the aerobic activity in the bench area.

Rope Jumping

Rope jumping is an excellent conditioning activity and of course it's fun—both children and adults can enjoy it. There's certainly plenty of room for jumping rope in the park, and it provides a nice change from the other activities.

In case you've forgotten the rope jumping of your childhood—the skills involved, the variations, the singsong chants and verses—we include here some material to refresh your memory and to reintroduce you to the joys of jumping rope.

Kinds of Ropes

Most commercially prepared jump ropes are about ten feet long and have a handle on each end. Some are made so that a person can unscrew a handle, cut the rope to a size that is comfortable for the user, and replace the handle. Adults can use a commercial jump rope uncut or trimmed only slightly; for a child, more can be cut away. The English type of commercially prepared jump rope has ball bearings in the handles and is supposedly easier to turn. See for yourself if you like it or need it.

Another excellent source of rope is your local hardware store. Heavy clothesline, known as no. 9 or no. 10 rope, comes in fifty-foot reels. That's enough rope for a family of five, at a fraction of the cost of commercial jump ropes. Your hardware store may also sell the rope by the foot, and this may be the cheapest way to buy one or two jump ropes.

A rough approximation of a comfortable length for jumping is double the distance from your shoulders to the floor. Drape the rope around your neck and cut it so that each end dangles about one half inch from the floor. Try jumping with this rope, winding it once around each hand for a comfortable hold. Adjust length as needed.

Some hardware stores carry only the light-weight clothesline rope known as no. 6 rope. Such rope is really too light for jumping, but you can use a reel of it to make one rope, beautifully weighted for jumping. The job, which requires only a simple chain stitch, is easy to do and will take less than an hour of your time.

We prefer a chain-stitched rope to a heavy no. 10 rope.

Directions for a chain-stitched rope are as follows (see diagrams on pages 138-39):

1. Cut about ten feet of rope from a fifty-foot reel of no. 6 rope. Trim it to double the distance from your shoulders to the floor. Jump with it, and shorten it if necessary for comfortable jumping. Use the resulting rope as your *guide rope*.
2. Make a simple loop nine or ten inches from one end of the rope (A). Cross the rope at the bottom of the loop.

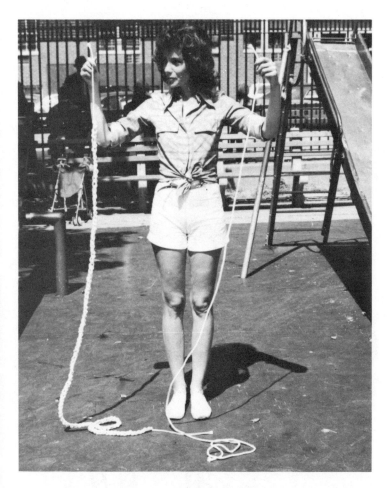

3. Make another loop from the long end near the first loop (B).
4. Push the second loop through the back of the first loop.
5. Place one hand on the short end of the rope and the other hand through the second loop. Tug so that the first loop forms a knot around the second loop (C). This is the basic chain stitch.

6. Continue the procedure, making a loop from the long end of the rope, pushing this loop through the preceding loop (D), and tugging to tighten. The chain stitch considerably shortens the rope and makes it very weighty. You need approximately forty feet of rope to make a ten-foot chain-stitched rope. Continue to the length of your guide rope and stop there.

7. For the last stitch, pull all the remaining rope through the last loop. Cut off all but about ten inches of the plain rope—enough to wind about your hand when jumping (E).

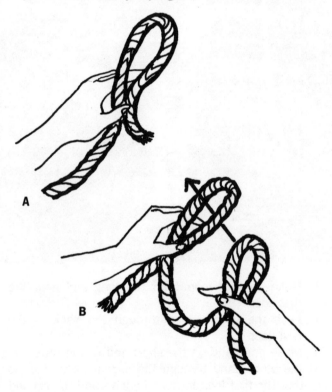

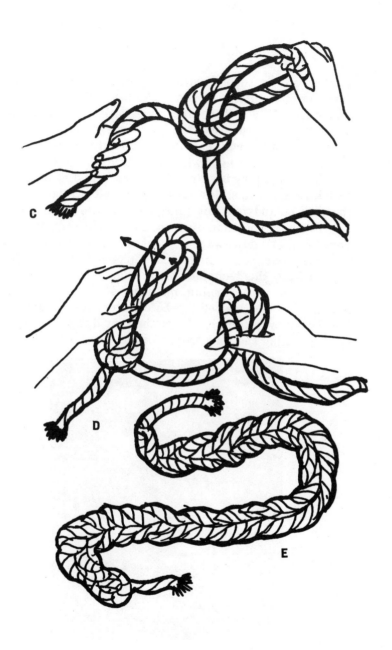

Turning the Rope

The rope is turned with a relaxed, easy wrist-and-forearm motion, elbows bent. The bent elbows are very important. If you turn the rope with arms extended straight, it is true that the rope will go higher above your head, but it will also hit the ground too far in front of you, and it will not swing clear below your feet.

Begin jumping in starting position: standing straight, feet together, arms close to the body, elbows bent. Hold the rope behind you, not quite touching the ground (A).

From this position, turn the rope backwards, up over your head, and downward in front of you. As the rope approaches your feet, jump so that it passes below you (B).

Practice this technique before you go on to any more complicated rope turning methods, such as the *Cross Swing* (crossing your elbows before every jump and opening them as you jump) (C), or the very difficult *Reverse Gear* (turning the rope from front to back).

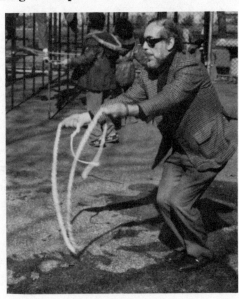

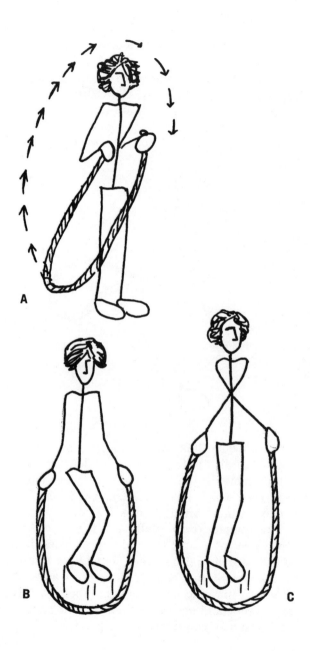

A

B

C

141

Basic Steps

There are three basic rope jumping steps: the One Step, the Simple Jump, and the Double Jump.

The One Step is not a jump but a leap in place. Start with one foot in the air, leap over the approaching rope onto the other foot, and so on, alternating feet (A). If

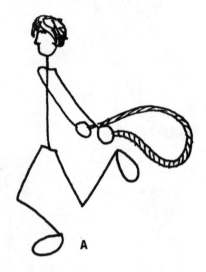

you haven't done this step in a long time, don't worry. It comes back quickly. If you've never done the One Step (if that's possible, if you grew up some place out in space), it may take a few days to learn, but it shouldn't be too difficult, even at an adult age.

The Simple Jump really is easy. You simply jump on both feet each time the rope approaches, keeping feet together. For a real beginner, it may be easier to learn than the One Step. The only things to watch out for are timing and jumping high enough (about two inches) to clear the rope and not tangle it with your feet. Again, the Simple Jump is just a matter of practice.

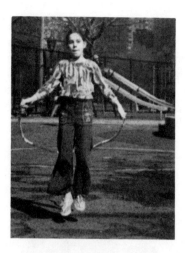

The Double Jump involves jumping to a different rhythm: two jumps for every turn of the rope. Jump two or three inches off the ground as the rope passes below you and about one inch off the ground as the rope peaks above you. Your jumping rhythm thus becomes a double beat with the first beat accented: JUMP, jump, JUMP, jump, JUMP.... It shouldn't take you long to master this step. Of the three basic steps described here, we prefer the Double Jump as the most vigorous conditioning activity.

There are many interesting variations on these three basic steps, and we shall describe some of them here. There is a valid reason for including this material in an exercise book. If you're interested, enjoying yourself, and physically active at the same time, that is, after all, what exercise is all about. You will probably find jumping rope much less boring than running in place in your bedroom. Also, no matter how old you are, it's still exciting to learn a new skill. So here is more material to challenge you and to challenge your children. These variations are more difficult than the basic steps and should be tried only after you have mastered the basics.

The **Cross Foot** is a variation of the Simple Jump. Cross your feet on one jump and uncross them on the next jump. Continue crossing and uncrossing your feet on alternate jumps.

The **Stork** is a variation of the One Step. Hop on one foot for five turns of the rope and then hop on the other

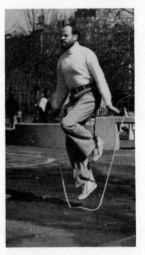

foot for five turns. Continue alternating feet every five turns.

The **Simple Spread** is another variation of the Simple Jump. Start with feet together, as in the Simple Jump, but at each jump increase the distance between your feet by a few inches until your legs are as far apart as they can be and still allow you to jump rope.

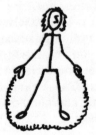

The **Double Spread** is similar to the Simple Spread but uses the rhythm of the Double Jump. As in the Simple Spead. Start with feet together and spread them farther and farther apart with each jump. The Double Spread is much more difficult than the Double Jump, but that only makes it more of a challenge!

The **Wooden Kick** is like the One Step except that you keep your legs stiff as you jump. Throw your raised leg forward and over the rope without bending the knee.

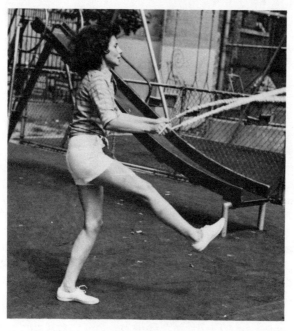

The technique is a series of forward kicks with alternate feet, something like a goose step. See how high you can kick without interfering with the turning rope.

Rope Jogging is the ideal conditioning activity. It combines the advantages of both jogging and rope jumping. Simply jump the rope while jogging at a comfortable pace. Establish your jogging rhythm as you move for-

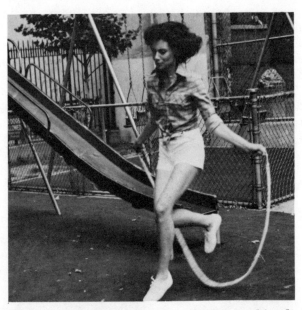

ward and then work the turning rope into this rhythm. This step is not for beginners.

When you can do all these basic steps and variations, then try to do them in Reverse Gear (turning the rope backwards.) If you can do that, you're a master and deserve a black belt or some other accolade in rope jumping!

Since this is something of a rope-jumping refresher, we want to remind you that there are very many activities and games that can be done while jumping rope. One such game is "Visiting." One person turns and jumps, and another person jumps in. The two people stand face to face and jump the same rope. This is an ideal game for a parent and a young child. The parent can pace the rope according to the child's age, agility, and coordination. Young children are usually delighted with this game and feel quite proud of their achievement when they first begin to jump.

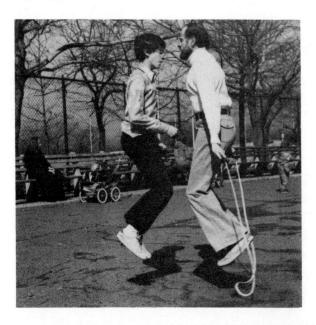

In another rope-jumping activity, two people called the *enders* turn the rope and a third person jumps in, usually with a singsong chant, and then jumps out. A variation for younger children is called "Baby's Cradle."

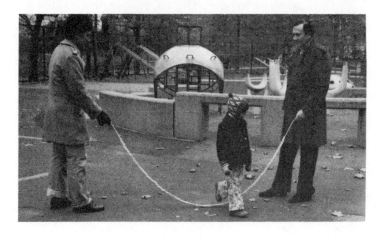

Instead of turning the rope, the enders sway the rope
from side to side low enough so that even very young
children can jump. You'll tire of this one long before the
children do. Even toddlers are fascinated with it. You can
adapt some of the songs and rhymes of rope jumping to
the rhythm of the swaying rope. These chants in themselves are—enchanting!

Remember this chant of middle childhood?

Teddy Bear, Teddy Bear, turn around.
Teddy Bear, Teddy Bear, touch the ground.
Teddy Bear, Teddy Bear, tie your shoe.
Teddy Bear, Teddy Bear, now skiddoo.

The person jumping acts out the chant and then
jumps out on the word *skiddoo*.

Or remember this one?

Mother, Mother, I am able
To cook the food and set the table.
Daughter, daughter, don't forget
Salt, vinegar, mustard, pepper.

On the word *pepper*, the rope is turned faster and
faster until the jumper stumbles or jumps out.

And do you recall this traditional welcome for a new
arrival?

Judge, Judge, tell the Judge.
Mama has a newborn baby.
It's not a girl.
It's not a boy.
It's just a newborn baby.
Wrap it up in tissue paper.
Send it down the elevator.
Third floor, pass; second floor, pass;
    first floor, OUT.

The amazing thing about these rhymes is that they are passed on from older children to younger children; they are part of the culture of childhood. We hear with astonishment today's children repeating rhymes and chants that evoke memories of our own childhood. Remember this one?

Cinderella, dressed in yeller,
Went downtown to meet her feller.
How many kisses did he give her?
One, two, three, four...

And the last number before the jumper stumbles reveals her fate.

And here was some rather rude advice to the older generation:

I like coffee, I like tea,
I like the boys and the boys like me.
Tell your mother to hold her tongue,
For she did the same when she was young.
Tell your father to do the same,
For he was the one who changed her name.

And to bring out the gypsy spirit in every child, the future is divined by rope jumping and stumbling! The verses are repeated until the player stumbles, and the word on which he stumbles is the key word that reveals, like a magic mirror in a fairy tale, what the future will be.

For example, about the husband-to-be and his occupation, we have this verse:

Rich man, poor man, beggar man, thief;
Doctor, lawyer, Indian chief;
Tinker, tailor, cowboy, sailor;
Butcher, baker, undertaker.

And his name?

Gypsy, gypsy, please tell me
What my husband's name will be?
A, B, C, D...

The letter called out before the player stumbles is
the first letter of her future husband's name.

And the wedding ceremony?

Where will we get married?
Church, synagogue, house, barn,
Church, synagogue, house...

The number of children?

How many children will we have?
One, two, three, four...

And finally, the heart of the matter!

Will he love me?
Yes, no, yes, no, yes...

And how about this one for crass materialism?

I should worry, I should care,
I should marry a millionaire.
He should die and I should cry,
And I should marry another guy.
How many husbands shall I have?
One, two, three, four, five, six...

Not every chant was about the future. If you grew
up in Depression or post-Depression days, you may remember that telephone calls were expensive and avoided
if possible. Some neighbors solved the problem by open-

ing their windows and carrying on conversations across rooftops or city streets—a habit that was reflected in the following rope-jumping chant:

My mother and your mother
Live across the street;
Last night they had a fight,
And this is what they said:

Icky bicky soda cracker
Icky bicky boo
Icky bicky soda cracker
Out goes you.

And do you recall this mysterious model of etiquette?

I am a little Dutch girl dressed in blue;
And these are the things I like to do:
Salute to the captain; bow to the queen.
And turn my back on the submarine!

Or this one?

"Hello, hello, hello, sir."
"Meet me at the grocer."
"No sir."
"Why sir?"
"Because I have a cold, sir."
"Where did you get your cold, sir?"
"At the North Pole, sir."
"What were you doing there, sir?"
"Shooting polar bear, sir."
"Let me hear you sneeze, sir."
"Kachoo, kachoo, kachoo, sir."

There are many other such verses and chants which belong to the folklore of childhood and which we include here to get you into the mood of rope jumping and the spirit of childhood. Remember Charley?

Charley over the water,
Charley over the sea.
Charley caught a blackbird,
But he can't catch me.

At the word *me*, the rope is turned faster and faster until the jumper stumbles or jumps out.

And doesn't everyone remember miming Dolly Dimple?

Dolly Dimple walks like this.
Dolly Dimple talks like this.
Dolly Dimple throws a kiss.
Dolly Dimple MISSES like this.

And the endless Michael Finnegan?

I know a man named Michael Finnegan.
He had whiskers on his chinnegan.
Along came a wind and blew them in again.
Poor old Michael Finnegan. Begin again.

These are all chants that were sung while two people turned the rope and the others jumped in and out. One parent alone can play in this way with young children in the park by tying one end of the rope to a fence and turning the other end while the children jump. It may be great fun for the children. For you, it's arm and shoulder exercise and also, we hope, fun. You can vary the exercise by turning with your left hand if you are right handed or vice versa. You can also vary it for everyone by sometimes turning clockwise and sometimes counterclockwise and also by very gradually raising the rope so that players have to jump higher and higher to clear it.

And finally there's Double Dutch, the game of champions! Two people (could be parents) work together to turn two ropes at the same time, one clockwise and the other, counterclockwise. The ropes turn like the interlocking cogs of a machine, and jumping them requires twice the speed and more than twice the skill needed for ordinary rope jumping. But this is already the higher mathematics of rope jumping, and we are concerned here only with the simple arithmetic.

Just keep in mind that rope jumping is a good conditioning activity for the cardiovascular system if done long enough and intensely enough to raise the pulse rate and, in a sense, exercise the heart muscle directly. From here on we invite you to explore on your own with your children and gain triple benefits: enjoyment, a shared experience, and a better level of physical fitness.

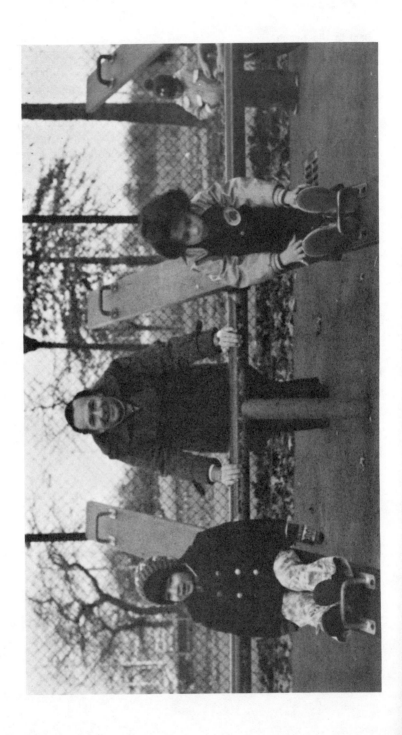

Chapter 9

The Individualized Approach

Some people prefer to be told precisely what to do: "Do these ten exercises, twenty-five minutes a day; just follow the directions exactly." In a way this approach seems simple. Do what you're told and you will achieve something known as "physical fitness." We think that's a sales spiel. It may be easy to sell such a program, but, in practice, that same kind of program will soon be dropped for a variety of reasons, not the least of which is boredom.

We believe that an exercise program should be tailor-made. Our needs are different; our bodies are different; our interests are different. We don't all dress alike. Why should our exercise programs be identical? On a recent trip to Peking, Bill Kovach wrote (*New York Times*, December 1, 1975):

In the early morning coalsmoke on these chill winter days the people of Peking appear to gather randomly at squares and on corners to practice wu-chu, a highly stylized ballet-like system of careful exercises.

Singly or in groups of 20 or more, blue-jacketed or gray-jacketed men and women, seemingly lost within themselves, work ever so correctly through the movements to bring head, arms, trunk and legs to the proper stance to conclude the exercise.

It staggers the imagination to think that millions of Chinese people, dressed alike, may be going through the same exercise movements every morning!

We believe that an individualized approach to exercise is the most valid one. You can be your own authority if you are informed and understand what you are doing. If you keep in mind the concept of a well-rounded exercise program outlined in Chapter 3 and understand the different goals of the various exercise philosophies, there is no reason why you can't design your own program to meet your own needs. Furthermore, you can change your program when your goals have been reached, or when your needs change, or when you begin to get bored with it. That is why we hope you will view this book, not as a series of rules and recipes to be followed rigidly, but rather as a source book of information and material that you can consult in planning your own individualized program.

You don't have to be a parent to use the playground for exercise. You can do all of the bench exercises, the seesaw slantboard exercises, and the jungle gym exercises alone, even without a child—provided, of course, that you are not usurping equipment from a child. (You can also do a friend a favor and take a friend's child to the playground, or a niece or a nephew.) The basic philosophy and approach of this book can be adapted to any environment. Once you begin to think about exercise creatively and to think of your own needs and goals also, you are not bound by any book or limited by any time or place. You can practice jogging anywhere; yoga-type exercises can be done in many different situations; isometrics, wherever you want to. About half of the exercises in this book can be adapted to different situations. You simply need to know yourself, to understand the goals of different types of exercise, and then to select suitable exercises to meet your own needs and goals. You can be your own expert.

The specific message that we have for parents of young children is the idea of working parallel with your child. Parallel play is a concept that has implications for many facets of parent-child relationships. For example, if a parent enjoys books, reads a great deal himself, and reads to children with obvious pleasure and satisfaction, those children will grow up reading and caring about books. It's that simple. Children have a way of knowing how an adult actually feels about a situation. If adults take the playtime at the park seriously, children will know this and not sense that subtle disregard for their play that sometimes, even unintentionally, is communicated to them.

Parents who go to the playground with their children have a great advantage in using the parallel play approach to the problem of exercise. The time is already

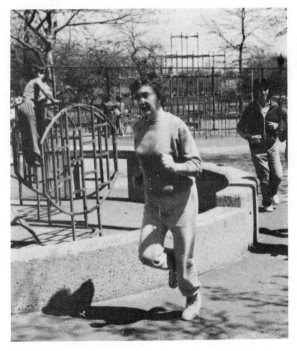

there; the place is already there; the habit pattern of going to the park is already established. All the parent has left to do is to make exercising part of this habit pattern and to enjoy doing so. In starting an exercise program, your first battle is already won by the fact that you have the time and the place set.

Since you have won the first battle without even trying, we suggest that you now sit down and roughly plan your schedule, taking into account your child's interests and usual activities at the playground, your own needs and goals, and the concept of what makes up a well-rounded exercise program. We have indexed the exercises in this book in a way that will make it easy for you to find quickly those exercises best suited to your needs. (See Index of Exercises). We suggest that your program include all four kinds of activities: yoga, isometrics,

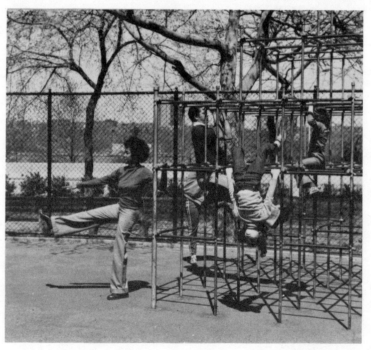

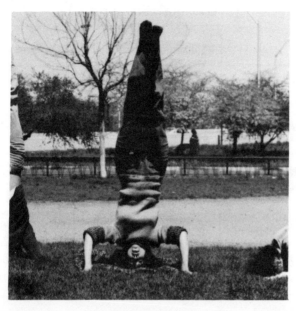

calisthenics, and aerobics. Don't forget that the calisthenic exercises, if done fast enough and long enough, can
qualify as conditioning exercises for the cardiovascular
system. If you use calisthenics in this way, you need not
add an aerobic activity. Our basic premise all along has
been that you can work this kind of program into your
regular daily excursions to the playground.

We suggest that in the beginning you concentrate on
six to eight exercises that you feel fit your needs and
your child's activities. To attempt to do all the exercises
in this book at once would be as foolish as going into a
restaurant and attempting to sample every item on the
menu. In fact, we could expand the analogy a bit and say
that what we are presenting here is an à la carte menu
of more than sixty playground exercises from which you
can select your own well-balanced and enjoyable exercise
"meal."

A sample selection might be as follows:

Exercise Schedule Form

	Apparatus	Page No.	Target
Warm-up *Acceler-ated bench walk*	Bench	36	Cardiovascular warm-up
Yoga-type exercises *The complete stretch*	Swings	62	Loosening up muscles, joints
Isometrics *The imaginary chair*	Jungle gym	94	Abdomen
Calisthenics *See-saw sit-up; see-saw push-up*	Seesaw	77 84	Abdomen, upper thighs; upper arms shoulders, abdomen
Aerobics Rope jumping	Bench or anywhere	135	Cardiovascular conditioning

Use the blank forms to make your own selections.

It is not even absolutely necessary to write down the exercises ahead of time. But in your own mind, at least, select the exercises that you want to work on; be aware of the goals that you want to reach; be flexible enough to change according to the availability of playground equipment and the needs of your own child. We hope it will soon become second nature to you to take advantage of your playground opportunities for parallel play exercise. We do not believe that you have to follow this or any other exercise book from A to Z in order to benefit.

We hope that you will select and use only those activities described here that you feel will contribute to the fulfillment of your own needs and goals. If you enjoy playing parallel at the playground with your child, and if you become more physically fit in the process, then this book will have served its intended purpose.

Exercise Schedule Form

	Apparatus	Page No.	Target
Warm-up			
Yoga-type exercises			
Isometrics			
Calisthenics			
Aerobics			

Exercise Schedule Form

	Apparatus	Page No.	Target
Warm-up			
Yoga-type exercises			
Isometrics			
Calisthenics			
Aerobics			

Exercise Schedule Form

	Apparatus	Page No.	Target
Warm-up			
Yoga-type exercises			
Isometrics			
Calisthenics			
Aerobics			

Exercise Schedule Form

	Apparatus	Page No.	Target
Warm-up			
Yoga-type exercises			
Isometrics			
Calisthenics			
Aerobics			

Bibliography

Abrahams, Roger D. *Jump-Rope Rhymes, A Dictionary.*
Austin: University of Texas Press, 1969.

Ald, Roy. *Jogging, Aerobics and Diet.* New York: Signet
Books, 1968.

Brown, Roscoe C., and Kenyon, Gerald D., eds. *Classical
Studies on Physical Activity.* Englewood Cliffs, N.J.:
Prentice-Hall, 1968.

Bucher, Charles A. *Foundations of Physical Education.*
St. Louis: C. V. Mosby, 1964.

Bucher, Charles A. "You Still Need Exercise." *Today's
Health* 34 (Dec. 1956), 12:24, 25, 56, 57, 58.

Cooper, Kenneth H., MD. *The New Aerobics.* New York:
Bantam Books, 1970.

Cooper, Kenneth H., MD. *Aerobics.* New York: Bantam
Books, 1968.

Cooper, Mildred, and Cooper, Kenneth H., MD. *Aerobics
for Women.* New York: Bantam Books, 1973.

Gawer, Herman, and Michelman, Herbert. *Body Control
and Physical Fitness.* New York: Crown, 1964.

Ginott, Haim. *Between Parent and Child.* New York:
Macmillan, 1965.

Gross, Leonard, and Morehouse, Lawrence E. *Total Fitness in 30 Minutes a Week.* New York: Simon &
Schuster, 1975.

Guidelines for Successful Jogging. Washington, D.C.:
The National Jogging Association, 1970.

Harris, W. E., and Bowerman, William J. *Jogging.* New York: Grosset & Dunlap, 1967.

Hittleman, Richard. *Yoga 28 Day Exercise Plan.* New York: Workman, 1969.

Jewett, Ann E., and Nixon, John E. *An Introduction to Physical Education.* Philadelphia: W. B. Saunders Co., 1969.

Johnson, Barry L., and Boudreaux, Patricia Duncan. *Basic Gymnastics for Girls and Women.* New York: Appleton-Century-Crofts, 1971.

Logan, Gene, and Wallis, Earl. *Figure Improvement and Body Conditioning.* Englewood Cliffs, N.J.: Prentice-Hall, 1964.

Luby, Sue. *Yoga Is for You.* Englewood Cliffs, N.J.: Prentice-Hall, 1974.

Moore, Marcia, and Douglas, Mark. *Yoga: Science of the Self.* York Cliffs, Maine: Arcane Books, 1967.

Nottidge, Pamela, and Lamplugh, Diana. *Slimnastics.* Baltimore: Penguin Books, 1973.

Patterson, Ann, and Halberg, Edmond C. *Background Readings for Physical Education.* New York: Holt, Rinehart and Winston, 1965.

Royal Canadian Air Force Exercise Plans for Physical Fitness. Rev. ed. Ottawa, Canada: Crown, 1962.

Shipley, Joseph T. *Dictionary of Word Origins.* Paterson, N.J.: Littlefield, Adams, & Co., 1961.

Skolnick, Peter L. *Jump Rope!* New York: Workman, 1974.

Tegner, Bruce. *Kung Fu and Tai Chi.* New York: Bantam Books, 1968.

Van Dalen, Deobold B.; Mitchell, Elmer D.; and Bennett, Bruce L. *World History of Physical Education.* Englewood Cliffs, N.J.: Prentice-Hall, 1960.

Withers, Carl, ed. *A Rocket in My Pocket.* New York: Holt, Rinehart and Winston, 1948.

Worstell, Emma V., ed. *Jump the Rope Jingles.* New York: Macmillan, 1961.

Index
to Exercises

INDEX (continued)

Name of Exercise	Apparatus*	Page	Basic Class**	Target
Leg Stretch	Jungle Gym	101	Yoga	thighs, flexible spine
Knee Hug	Swing	52	Calisthenics	lower back, thighs
Palm Tree	Swing	50	Yoga	thighs, balance
Posture Improver	Jungle Gym	95	Isometrics	pelvic alignment, abdomen
Rag Doll Shakes	Bench (A)	35	Calisthenics	limbering up
Rope Jumping	Rope	135	Aerobics	cardiovascular conditioning
Seesaw Back Kick	Seesaw	70	Hybrid—Calisthenics/Yoga	arms, legs
Seesaw Cat	Seesaw	85	Yoga	upper arms, shoulders, spine
Seesaw Jog	Seesaw	72	Aerobics	cardiovascular conditioning
Seesaw Pump	Seesaw	67	Hybrid—Yoga/Calisthenics	thighs, back
Seesaw Push-up	Seesaw	84	Calisthenics	upper arms, shoulders, abdomen
Seesaw Sit-up	Seesaw	77	Calisthenics	abdomen, upper thighs
Seesaw Squat	Seesaw	69	Calisthenics	arms, legs, thighs
Seesaw Twist	Seesaw	73	Yoga	waist
Serpent	Seesaw	83	Yoga	lower back
Side Jogging	Swing	60	Aerobics	cardiovascular conditioning
Side Lift	Seesaw	86	Yoga	abdomen, hips, thighs
Side Swing Stretch	Swing	44	Hybrid—Calisthenics/Yoga	thighs, waist
Sky Stretch	Swing	53	Yoga	relaxation of muscles, joints
Spinal Stretch	Bench (A)	133	Yoga	thighs, spine
Swing Squat	Swing	58	Hybrid—Calisthenics/Yoga	lower back, thighs, balance

*The letter (A) after the name of the apparatus denotes that the exercise is easily adaptable to other apparatus in the playground.

**Here we identify the basic type of exercise. An exercise classified as "Yoga" may not be identical to a yoga exercise, but it may be derived from a yoga exercise, and its main feature is stretching and holding. "Calisthenics" means the main benefit is strengthening and toning of muscles through repetitive movement. Exercises designated "Isometrics" strengthen the muscles without movement. "Aerobics" means the main benefit is the strengthening of the cardiovascular-respiratory system. Some exercises may be "Hybrid," e.g., a combination of yoga and calisthenics; the first mentioned class is the dominant one. It is understood that, if calisthenics are done at a fast pace, they have aerobic qualities; while, if they are done at a slow pace with stretching and holding, they have yoga qualities.